HEALTHCARE SOCIAL MEDIA

Transformation 3.0

*Dynamic, Cutting-Edge, Results-Oriented
Communication 2015 and Beyond*

GARY W. LAWSON, DPA

ISBN: 1505541719
ISBN 13: 9781505541717
Library of Congress Control Number: 2014922680
CreateSpace Independent Publishing Platform

North Charleston, South Carolina

TABLE OF CONTENTS

PREFACE

HEALTHCARE PROVIDERS WHO are able to transform their organizations to incorporate social media and other emerging technologies will thrive and prosper in the new healthcare environment.

Social media permeates every facet of our lives. Social media and rapid technological advancements are here, and they are quickly evolving. These changes can't be ignored. No matter how much healthcare providers want to, they can't fight the exponential changes in technology; there is no turning back the clock. Using Internet tools for healthcare communication and information management offers a tremendous opportunity for providers to expand their mission to further help their patients. No one knows for sure what the healthcare industry of the future will look like, but healthcare innovators will be using social media and new technologies that will reinvent healthcare best practices as we know them.

Healthcare providers are caring professionals who constantly communicate with patients, their families, and their peers. It is inevitable that as social media continues to become an integral part of everyday communication, providers must acquire new virtual communication skills and use new digital communication methodologies.

The healthcare industry faces considerable challenges arising from different issues. Such chaotic changes call for strong, clinically based leadership and good governance to address the ever-evolving healthcare needs of patients, government regulations, and payers across the United States.

Today's best practices are evolving in terms of patient communication and managing patient outcomes. In most healthcare journals, what is commonly mentioned in terms of leadership is transformational or charismatic leadership. This type of leadership can motivate, educate, inspire, and encourage members of the healthcare provider team to achieve better organizational outcomes.

To promote patient-centered care, healthcare providers must promote staff empowerment and patient involvement. The form of communication used today is no longer from top to bottom; rather, it is a conversation between patients and their providers. Now is the time for Healthcare Social Media Transformation 3.0, in which engaged patients become better informed and make better healthcare choices.

Healthcare providers are embracing collaborative work among and between other disciplines in the provision of holistic patient care. The management of care is now composed of expert personnel and providers from various specialties working together to meet or improve the patient's outcome. Healthcare providers are continuously coordinating and sharing information with other members of the team to provide excellent patient-centered care to every patient in the system.

Going forward, providers must maximize their use of modern technology as a reliable partner to improve the quality of care, accuracy, safety, and efficiency to patients and the workforce. The full use of electronic data in recording the patient's progress and in the reimbursement process from third-party providers illustrates just two of the new changes in the management and leadership style being utilized today.

As healthcare moves to an evidence-based modality, providers are expected to offer patient care at a more affordable cost. For the healthcare industry to maximize patient outcomes, reduce costs, and increase organizational success, providers will need to continually reevaluate their roles professionally, increase their use of new technologies, and unceasingly envision and use new virtual communication methodologies to shape the provider-patient experience.

This book discusses a variety of social media tools and explains how they are being used in healthcare to maximize quality of care, improve patient outcomes, expand communication and collaboration, and increase profits.

1

SOCIAL MEDIA IS
TRANSFORMING
HEALTHCARE

THE USE OF social media is growing exponentially. Millions of people go online each day to seek healthcare information, do research, post updates, share photos, write and read blogs, locate and review healthcare providers, watch videos, play games, and more. Social media sites attract people from every demographic. Due to social media's expanding popularity and opportunities, many healthcare businesses have created an online presence.

Social networks are becoming increasingly important in healthcare. For example, the Centers for Disease Control and Prevention (CDC) uses social networks to share timely, accurate health information. During the 2009 flu season, CDC YouTube views reached 2.6 million, podcast downloads totaled 1.5 million, and the CDC's Facebook followers totaled more than 55,000. The CDC's H1N1 website had more than 200 million page views, and its emergency profile on Twitter was tracked by 1.2 million followers.[1] Social media played a vital role during the flu epidemic because people were looking for information on a cure, the signs of symptoms, disease management, and other details that could help them make better healthcare choices.

Social media takes the mystery out of healthcare information. Healthcare authority sites, like WebMD and the Mayo Clinic, translate their articles into terms that can be easily understood by the general public. Healthcare professionals are also including animations, infographics, videos, and photos. By incorporating visual communications with easy-to-understand written information, healthcare professionals are creating more opportunities for patient participation and involvement.

Healthcare social media sites give millions of people an opportunity to share their experience, knowledge, understanding, support, compassion, and expertise regarding their medical conditions. One example developed by the American Cancer Society is the Cancer Survivors Network. The primary purpose of this network, as it is for many patient-to-patient platforms, is peer support.[2]

The growing popularity of social media allows more Americans to obtain online information regarding specific therapies and healthcare conditions. Likewise, healthcare providers use social networks for professional purposes, including collaboration and information gathering.

Social media connects people from all walks of life without regard to ethnicity, economics, religion, political affiliation, age, gender, or race. It allows patients to interact with each other through forums, blogs, instant messaging, comments, and virtual video chats. In other words, social networking platforms give patients the opportunity to support, connect, educate, and empower one another more than at any other time in history.

According to a recent Pew survey:[3]

- Thirty-three percent of American adults have used the web to research a medical issue.
- Fifty-one percent of people would feel more valued as a patient via digital health communications.
- Forty-one percent of people said that social media would affect their choice of healthcare providers.

- Fourteen percent (seven hundred out of more than five thousand) of the hospitals in the United States use social media. Hospitals use social networks for promotional purposes and to monitor consumers' experiences of the services they've received.
- Thirty-six percent of social-network users evaluate and leverage other consumers' knowledge before making healthcare decisions. Social networks offer organizations an opportunity to reach stakeholders, promote collaboration, and aggregate information. [4]

The biggest social media risk a hospital can take is to ignore social media. It seems as though hospitals are changing, as demonstrated in the 2014 Most Wired (i.e., highest users of social media) Survey:
(Why are the dots below smaller than the dots above?)

- Ninety-seven percent of hospitals using social media have Facebook, 83 percent have YouTube, 81 percent have Twitter, and 74 percent have LinkedIn.
- Ninety-eight percent of the hospitals on social media use it to disseminate information, 94 percent to give updates on hospital events, and 91 percent to update the public on service lines. In addition, 96 percent use social media for community engagement, and 77 percent use it for patient education.

While the majority of all hospitals seem to be doing a good job of starting to use social media for outgoing information, few hospitals use it for patient engagement. Only 22 percent use social media to livestream procedures or surgeries. According to the Most Wired Survey, only 33 percent of hospitals surveyed use social media to connect primary care physicians with specialty services within the health system. [5]

Potential Drawbacks of Using Healthcare Social Media

Obviously, Health Insurance Portability and Accountability Act (HIPAA) regulations come into play with healthcare social media—as do legitimate concerns about data hacking. Still, social media can be a powerful tool to educate physicians not just within the confines of a single physical location, but around the world. Telemedicine is already helping physicians connect with one another as well as patients.

The Internet, of course, has no overseeing authority that audits and counterchecks the accuracy of information. Therefore, as social media networks bridge the patient/provider relationship gap, this new form of communication is vulnerable to computer hackers, identity thieves, and other con artists posing as healthcare experts.

Despite state-of-the-art firewalls and security, social media sites and organizations are vulnerable to scammers who can extract data or shut down a system to satisfy their own interests. Providers should avoid open, public social media channels to communicate with patients and one another, even when sending private messages. In all cases, HIPAA laws must be upheld to protect the confidentiality of patient information.

While social media offers communication platforms for patient advocacy, they are also an easy way to spread negative feedback, especially from dissatisfied patients or disgruntled workers within the organization. These situations must be addressed quickly, unemotionally, and professionally. Social media should always be managed by a communications plan that specifically outlines employee social behavior and etiquette on the Internet. To minimize the loss of employee productivity, organizations should have a written policy that regulates the use of social media during work hours.

Ongoing monitoring of social media allows organizations to be proactive and minimize the spread of negative information. Both negative and positive feedback offer valuable information that can help healthcare leaders improve products and services. Gathered feedback can also serve as an evaluation and satisfaction tool that can be used to make positive changes in patients' experiences.

Social Media for Healthcare Research
Healthcare agencies that do research are now using social media platforms. These sites allow researchers to expand their studies at a very low cost. Research studies are often done on blogs and

healthcare authority sites by offering surveys or sending invitations to join an online discussion group.

Social Media Connects Healthcare Providers

Clinicians are using social media to connect with other professionals. The Health5C website, which claims to be the largest online community of doctors, allows clinicians to find and connect with colleagues to securely share information. The privacy of the site is maintained as users are validated and checked. Provider-to-provider social media sites support confidential information sharing and virtual collaboration. The American Medical Association (AMA) and American Nurses Association (ANA) have issued comprehensive social media guidelines for their members, and other organizations are starting to do the same.

In September 2011 QuantiaMD performed a study entitled "Doctors, Patients & Social Media." It explored the relevance of social media in healthcare and, more specifically, how clinicians use social media to improve the quality of healthcare. The responses of the 4,033 clinicians surveyed included the following:

- Twenty-eight percent of respondents already use professional physician communities to learn from experts and peers.
- There is a significant need for secure, convenient forms of electronic communication that clinicians can use to correspond with one another and with patients.
- Twenty percent of clinicians use two or more sites for personal and professional use; these "connected clinicians" are the most eager to use social media to improve healthcare.[6]

Improving Patient Health Outcomes

Many healthcare leaders are starting to use social media to engage potential patients and increase market share. Marketing is one of many ways providers can use social media.

When a patient goes to a healthcare provider, the provider initiates a conversation and engages the patient to obtain the best outcome. Similarly, social media sites are designed to virtually engage consumers. Providers should use these new methodologies to virtually extend quality care that supports their patient long after the visit ends.

Social media can help providers educate, inform, inspire, mentor, and virtually assist their patients to make better healthcare decisions and obtain improved outcomes. By virtually increasing quality patient care, providers will receive more word-of-mouth referrals and higher pay-for-performance scores. [7]

Social media makes it easy for patients and physicians to connect outside the exam room. Therefore, primary care and other private-practice doctors are building an online presence. It's too soon to take for granted that a physician will be on Facebook or Twitter, but that could be the norm in a few years. More than a thousand doctors are registered with TwitterDoctors.net, a database of physicians who tweet. In fact, Emmy Award–winning medical journalist Dr. Sanjay Gupta can be found on Twitter (@DrSanjayGupta). "These are powerful, tremendously influential tools," says internist Kevin Pho of Nashua, New Hampshire, a popular medical blogger who engages with his patients via Facebook and Twitter. "Doctors should be taking advantage of the opportunity."[8]

Easier communication between healthcare providers and their patients will become a significant part of the quality patient experience. Patient engagement includes but is not limited to the following: providers talking to their patients and vice versa, patients talking to one another, and providers talking to other providers. Virtually extending care and initiating communication, information, support, inspiration, and education will be increasingly important as pay-for-performance comes into play in 2018. [9]

According to the PriceWaterhouse Coopers report cited in an article by John Trader, consumers trust social media from doctors more than they trust information from hospitals, health insurers, or drug companies. This indicates that clinicians still remain at the center of the communications model. [10]

The healthcare industry is in a major upheaval. With pay-for-performance mandates, the relationship between a provider and patient will likely become more profound and deep-rooted than a simple contractual relationship. Providers have traditionally been given more power and respect than other professionals, but the question remains: Can this critical relationship be extended virtually using social media to improve patient health outcomes?

More doctors and nurses are using Facebook, Twitter, and other platforms to interact with and monitor their patients. For example, Ruthi Moore, director of nursing for the Navy-Marine Corps Relief Society, monitors Afghanistan and Iraq veterans using Facebook. By keeping track of the updates, she can see when one of her clients starts to get depressed and suicidal. On more than one occasion, Ms. Moore learned of a potentially critical situation from Facebook updates, and she was able to intervene in time to help.

Monitoring social media offers additional benefits for patients who are isolated—geographically, mentally, medically, or all three. Counselors have helped returning service personnel, even those who are especially reluctant to ask for help. Moore and her fifty-two nurses, for instance, monitor their patients by creating professional Facebook and Twitter accounts. Then, they ask their patients to connect. Most of the veterans they treat will friend and follow them, and many then forget about it. So, most of the time, the interaction is passive. Some nurses post links regarding a new handbook or articles on a given health topic like nutrition or posttraumatic stress disorder; otherwise they keep an eye on Facebook updates using e-mail alerts that a friend has added a new post, video, or picture. [11]

Healthcare Social Media 2015

Is your healthcare organization suffering from fear of missing out, also known as FOMO? Are you wondering if other healthcare providers are getting more and/or better results using social media?

The Clinical Advisor's Social Media Survey shown on the chart below looks at social media use in 2015. Overall, 350 nurse practitioners and physician assistants responded to a survey in August and September 2014.

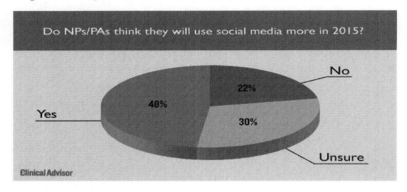

Understanding and using social media has many advantages for healthcare providers. After receiving real-time information about the marathon bombing from people on the scene tweeting, trauma teams in Boston were able to prepare for patients much sooner than if notice had come from traditional communication sources. Because of the real-time advantage of Twitter, surgeons were able to stop elective surgeries and prepare the rooms for people coming in from the bombing.[12]

Overworked healthcare providers can save the hours they spend teaching the same information over and over again by uploading a single YouTube video. Providers trying to explain a complicated health procedure to a patient can provide far more context, clarity, and help to expedite their conversation by referring the patient to a video, podcast, infographic, blog, or article ahead of time. If health-care providers give patients information in advance (e.g., podcast, YouTube video, etc.), they can begin the conversation at a higher level.

Social media has also empowered patients, especially those with truly unique conditions. Social media that is patient driven, not pro-vider driven, allows patients to have better insight into their own medical conditions. Even people who are isolated can now become an integral, active member of an online patient-to-patient support community.

In conclusion, social media holds a promising future for engaging patients and their families, thereby improving healthcare outcomes. At this time there are few, if any, proven best methods. However, social media sites are free and popular, and millions of people use them daily to get information. Healthcare providers need to engage their patients with valuable, relevant, open, and honest communication that creates solid, ongoing, virtual patient-provider relationships. Using social media to help patients obtain better health outcomes will always be a work in progress.

2

From Sledgehammer To Engagement

Traditional Healthcare Outbound Marketing 1.0

MANY HEALTHCARE PROVIDERS and organizations are comfortable using traditional, old-school marketing (outbound marketing) and conservative patient education. Old-school techniques focus on finding customers. However, these techniques are poorly targeted, expensive, inefficient, and designed to interrupt the target audience with a sales message. Traditionalists use print advertising, billboards, television/radio advertising, flyers, postcards, junk mail, spam, cold calls, trade shows, and many more promotional methods, hitting their key audience in the head with sledgehammer-type communication and marketing techniques.

Advances in technology and the Internet make outbound marketing communication techniques seem crude, out of date, less effective, and more expensive. Caller ID blocks cold calls. TiVo makes television advertising less effective. Spam filters block mass e-mails, and tools like Really Simple Syndication (RSS) make print and display advertising less useful. Regardless of the changes in technology, it is still possible to get a message out using older, more traditional methodologies, but it costs more and offers decreasing long-term value.

Healthcare Inbound Marketing Communication 2.0

Whether or not the healthcare industry is ready to change, inbound marketing—the opposite of outbound marketing—is quickly becoming the norm. Instead of hitting their general target market on the head with a sledgehammer, inbound marketers place their message where it can be found by specifically identified, targeted key publics. Instead of interrupting people with television ads, inbound marketers create videos that potential customers *want to see*. Instead of buying display ads in publications, inbound marketers create a business blog that key publics *want to read*. Instead of cold calling, inbound marketers create useful content and tools so that targeted individuals will contact the healthcare organization to *request more information*. Instead of driving a general message into a crowd over and over again like a sledgehammer, inbound marketers work hard to attract highly qualified customers.

Inbound 2.0 healthcare marketing communication campaigns have three key components:

> 1. **Relevant Content Creation and Dissemination**—This is the core of a healthcare, set-yourself-up-to-be-found, inbound marketing strategy. It is the dissemination of relevant information that attracts potential patients to click through to a website or use a business.

> 2. **Search Engine Optimization (SEO)**—SEO is the practice of maximizing a healthcare organization's priority ranking in search engines for targeted key words. SEO techniques make it easier for patients to find and use your services.

> 3. **Social Media Platforms**—Using social media increases the impact of a healthcare organization's communication. When content is distributed across and discussed on personal relationship networks, the communication becomes more trustworthy, and therefore, it is more likely to attract qualified patients to use healthcare products and services.

Healthcare Inbound 2.0 Marketing Communication Makes Sense

An increasing number of healthcare organizations are using inbound marketing because it is a more efficient, effective, and less expensive way to allocate limited marketing resources. When using inbound marketing, using common sense and creating relevant content are more important than spending more money pursuing outdated outbound marketing methodologies. In other words, in this new inbound 2.0 marketing environment, the capacity of the brain is more important than the size of the wallet.

Inbound marketing improves efficiency over traditional outbound marketing—and it costs less. Outbound marketing is about spending money, whereas inbound marketing is about creating content and spreading the word. Twitter, Facebook, Google+, and a blog are free to set up and only require time to start and maintain. These tools can attract the attention of potential patients by the thousands. Therefore, the return on investment (ROI) from inbound marketing is much higher than outbound marketing.

Traditional outbound marketing is poorly targeted, while inbound marketing is specifically targeted to people who demonstrate an interest in the content. These people are then more likely to be interested in specific healthcare products and services. Outbound marketing spends money. The advertisement or campaign is executed, and then it is gone, whereas inbound marketing sets up cumulative communication tools that continue to add value over time.

In the early days of the Internet, there was no mainstream healthcare inbound marketing. There were a lot of experiments, but few online healthcare business buyers and consumers. Inbound marketing tools and the public's use of them have evolved to the point where inbound marketing is now practical. In the mid-1990s, as the first Internet bubble grew, companies began to follow their customers online. At the beginning, healthcare businesses scattered advertising across mass media Internet sites in hopes of finding a few potential patients who would see the advertisements and respond.[13]

When the dot-com bubble broke in 2001, healthcare marketers began to reassess the effectiveness of scattering advertisements on popular Internet sites. They saw that other industries were purchasing fewer ads on mass media sites and spending more on pay-per-click ads on search engines. They soon discovered that, in many cases, targeted search engine advertising was far more effective than display advertising on mass media sites.

As more money was spent on search engine pay-per-click marketing, a new era of Internet growth began. This new phase, Web 2.0, produced significant changes in the way people viewed and used the Internet, which shifted from being a read-only experience to one in which everyone could publish, connect, and share online content.

Today's healthcare marketers are effectively using the tools of this new read-write web to become more efficient and effective. They are starting to become inbound marketing communication specialists, using social media to optimize content as a means to promote business. With the new inbound marketing tools becoming mainstream, the scale of healthcare business development can be unlimited. If the organization offers quality products and services and has the new inbound skills to communicate with its customers, it can successfully compete with the biggest advertising budgets. This shift to inbound 2.0 marketing communication is exciting and empowering for smaller healthcare businesses.

As the Internet moves into a 3.0 environment (personal identification, conversation, and engagement), the 2.0 social read-write environment continues. When Internet users could post information and transfer it from person-to-person, the 2.0 social connection was moved to online platforms. Starting with social websites like Friendster and Myspace, networks were created to connect people, see photos, get reminders on important dates, and much more. LinkedIn created a virtual business network, and Facebook, YouTube, Twitter, and Foursquare allow people to share their every move by video, photo, location check-in, and status update.

In 2.0 people friended or followed others the way they once searched for information and news using keywords. Facebook is the clear leader in 2.0, setting the standard for how relationships are measured. It has more than one billion users and is growing. YouTube is the video giant with more than one billion unique users monthly. Meanwhile, Twitter has carved out a solid and rapidly expanding niche for microblogging and real-time information, and Foursquare is the location innovator. But overall, Facebook dwarfs all competition and remains the reigning king of 2.0.[14]

Transformational Healthcare 3.0

Now that the world's information is posted, linked, indexed, and searchable—and people are connecting, sharing, liking, and following—it is time for the Internet to get another dimension. This new dimension is not measured by data or by which search engine led to these data. Internet 3.0 is about engaging the user as an individual. It is about each person's specific pursuits, wants, desires, preferences, and chosen engagement within narrow, specifically selected Internet niche environments.[15]

In addition to the increasing personalization of the Internet, 3.0 includes more mobile capabilities and geolocation opportunities. With smartphones and tablets becoming more prevalent and powerful, these new tools are becoming an extension of who people are as individuals. Also, mobile devices are being used more often to discover relevant information content, places, services, and products.

Some Internet providers say they are "personal" 3.0 when, in fact, most of what they do is "social" 2.0. These 2.0 services often use information gathered in the social experience to provide personalized recommendations based on what similar people may like. Some services say they are personal because people have specifically provided others with information about themselves and what they like. This information-gathering method is closer to discovering an individual's interests, but it is incomplete and, most likely, inaccurate due to the finite information given.

Beyond the 3.0 wannabes' initial attempts to make the Internet personal, there is a new wave of companies trying to crack the code of the "real you as an individual." My6sense.com and Gravity.com try to deliver a personalized experience in all possible aspects of an individual's life, finding the right information at the right time in the right context, based on that person's exact preferences.

Aside from My6sense and Gravity, there are other companies working to find the "real you." TiVo, Amazon, and Netflix are designed to give personal recommendations.[16] LinkedIn purchased mSpoke to provide personal recommendations,[17] and Facebook uses a new algorithm that chooses what it decides is the most important information for the individual user.[18]

As more companies switch to a 3.0 individualization and personalization of the Internet, it is exactly the right time for the healthcare industry to get on board. Healthcare is very personal; it is not a one-size-fits-all proposition. Patients are not like anyone else. Their interests are unique, and the status of their health is unique. Thus, with the rapid growth of accurate personal health information, healthcare information sharing, healthcare engagement, healthcare personalization, and healthcare persuasive connectivity—and with the increased capability and prevalence of smartphones and other mobile devices—it is time to create a virtual, extremely personal, effective 3.0 healthcare delivery enhancement system.

Healthcare 3.0 will help patients make better choices. It will inspire, educate, inform, mentor, monitor, and help them have a higher quality of life and achieve better health outcomes.

Social Media 3.0 Can Change Healthcare Behavior

The twenty-first century brought new healthcare communication and information possibilities. The rapidly evolving changes in technology made access to healthcare information much easier and faster. People across all age groups now use the Internet to search for healthcare information, connect to someone with the same healthcare issues, share information, and entertain themselves. Social media platforms have become increasingly popular with the masses.

In 2007, according to the Health Information National Trends Survey (HINTS), approximately 69 percent of adults were involved in different Internet activities such as blogging, visiting social media sites, and participating in online support groups. In other words, social media had already affected the majority of Americans as early as 2007. This study suggested that new technology and social media have been changing healthcare communication across the United States for many years. Access to information is instantaneous, which is why social media marketers have changed their traditional out-bound marketing model in order to compete.[19]

Patient-focused networks that concentrate on a specific disease or condition give individuals and their families an opportunity to receive comfort, insights, and potential leads on new treatments. These online communities encourage members to build relation-ships, share stories, and become more informed.

CureDiva (curediva.com)

CureDiva helps breast cancer patients and survivors. The site sells a large variety of products and gives its members suggestions and support from the online community of breast cancer survivors. Members can choose their privacy level and explore tips, blogs, discussion groups, and more. Providers who specialize in breast cancer treatment can give patients access to this and similar sites.

WEGO Health Network (wegohealth.com)

Designed for users who are actively involved in healthcare online, WEGO Health Network is a free social network where advocates connect, share experiences and advice, and get the press credentials required to cover many health conferences. Members can integrate their WEGO infor-mation with profiles from other social networks such as Twitter, Facebook, and LinkedIn to cross-promote articles or videos they create for WEGO. WEGO Health is a net-work of over one hundred thousand of the most influential members of the online health community and includes bloggers, tweeters, pinners, and leaders of Facebook pages. These are the empowered patients that drive the healthcare conversation online, across virtually every health topic and condition.

Information on health prevention and promotion is readily accessible online. The challenge, however, for both the healthcare industry and consumers is determining the accuracy of that information. The relationship between social media and improved health outcomes has produced the following conflicting results:

Positive
- Internet-based social networks can increase perceived social support and interconnectivity among individuals.
- With the increase of user-generated content, information sharing enables users to exchange health-related information, which makes the information more patient centered.
- Public health programs have successfully adopted social media as a communication platform for promoting such efforts as smoking cessation and dietary interventions.

Negative
- On social media there is always the possibility of widespread dissemination of potentially erroneous health information. Readers are cautioned to verify information before accepting it as fact.

Social Media in Healthcare: A Patient's Perspective

The diagnosis of a serious illness, whether it is life threatening like cancer or chronic like diabetes, can leave a person feeling isolated and lost. Often patients wonder why it has happened to them. Now, through a variety of social media and other online resources, a patient can find a way to cope with these challenges.

Through a website like CarePages, a family can create a blog and post updates on all that the patient is going through during treatment. Using this resource, family and friends all around the world can be kept informed without worrying about phone calls or e-mail. Then, patients can receive an enormous amount of support through the family and friends who visit their personal page, and supporters can post caring and supportive comments. Through social media resources, patients can also find other patients who are or were in a similar condition.

To help other teens dealing with and recovering from cancer, Clarissa Schilstra started www.teen-cancer.com in 2011 and continues to post on it today. While Clarissa set out to simply make it a resource for other young people going through cancer treatment, it has become very therapeutic for her. Writing blog posts has been a very positive experience because it has enabled her to process her journey through cancer treatment and life as a two-time cancer survivor.

After a devastating diagnosis, healthcare providers should tell patients about social media support sites. Social media resources can be very effective tools to help patients cope with their diagnoses as these outlets enable them to assist others going through similar healthcare experiences at similar stages in life. Additionally, such sites are much more flexible than structured support services, like support groups. Through these virtual methods, patients can connect with others who can understand what they are going through, even while being confined to a hospital bed or sofa at home. Patients can also choose to form support groups from those connections.

Healthcare 3.0 Looking toward the Future

Healthcare 3.0 offers real-time patient information, inspiration, and engagement. Many overworked healthcare providers are rolling their eyes right now at the thought of adding another layer of patient interaction to an already impossible schedule. However, helping a patient at the earliest possible time could reduce the severity of the problem, leading to a better healthcare outcome.

Healthcare Transformation 3.0 is a process, not a project. There is no end date. Unlike the time-restricted office visit, 3.0 is a

24/7/365 virtual, ongoing, and significant future best practice for providing quality, personalized care.

Too often today, patients are herded in and out of healthcare facilities. To extend quality care, providers need to offer the best possible virtual patient-centered care. This means increasing the influence of healthcare providers over patients virtually, long after the office visit ends. Healthcare 3.0 uses social media and other rapidly advancing technology to create a virtual patient-centered environment, providing more opportunities to maximize patient satisfaction and healthcare outcomes and increase pay-for-performance revenue.

Many organizations continually work to improve patient services and quality. It is important to keep in mind that the patient experience must extend beyond the office visit. Not only is a patient-centered focus the right thing to do, but reimbursement will partially be based on customer-satisfaction scores. Thus, providing excellent customer service can help drive revenue.

Within electronic medical records (EMRs) and practice-management systems, patient engagement is defined as tools and resources that help patients keep track of appointments, billing, health records, and test results.[21] It's important for providers and patients to be able to manage this information digitally, but there's so much more that is needed if providers want to improve health outcomes and make a positive impact. In my opinion, the new healthcare information technology (IT) systems are incapable of dramatically impacting patient behavior, especially regarding complex chronic conditions. By using social media and other advancing technologies in addition to IT solutions, providers can virtually engage their patients in the following ways (partial list):

1. **Educate Patients and Their Families**—Healthcare 3.0 can inform and educate patients and their families. With more relevant information, patients can have more meaningful discussions with friends, family, and healthcare professionals, which will help them make informed healthcare choices.

2. **Promote Personal Responsibility**—Healthcare 3.0 can monitor, inspire, encourage, and support positive patient healthcare behaviors and decisions.

3. **Encourage Proactive Care**—Healthcare 3.0 can help patients be more proactive in their own care and encourage them to meet their healthcare goals.

4. **Harness Self-Interest**—Healthcare 3.0 can help patients make conscious cost vs. value decisions based on targeted, relevant information.

Healthcare providers who use advancing technologies and a social media–based, virtual, patient-centered focus are more likely to flourish under the new Medicare requirements. To increase patient and family engagement, it will become increasingly important for providers to virtually communicate with their patients and families. Social media tools and cutting-edge technology will provide patients with appropriate real-time information about their conditions and methods of management. With the use of social media by the healthcare team, patients will be more aware, educated, informed, motivated, and empowered. Now is the time to use social media to help patients make better personal healthcare choices and to promote better patient outcomes.

3

HEALTHCARE PROMOTION

MARKETING IS ONLY one of many benefits that can be derived by using healthcare social technologies. Too often, healthcare organizations associate social media and other advancing technologies exclusively with marketing. Although social media can be used for marketing, businesses that harness and use new technologies for the many other possibilities will be the innovative, visionary businesses that reap the highest benefits and most of the profits.

In a changing healthcare environment, organizations are making important decisions about how to improve access to patient data using health information exchanges and online patient portals.[22] However, successfully engaging patients and meeting the new requirements may not be synonymous. To truly impact patient behavior and motivate positive health changes requires a comprehensive strategy for patient engagement that includes a strong virtual component.

New healthcare IT systems are simply not enough to impact individual patient behavior, especially for complex chronic conditions. Improved patient outcomes depend on higher levels of engagement, current and accurate information, and education and support provided to the patient virtually on an ongoing basis. Using social media to engage patients offers providers the opportunity to stay in virtual contact with them to educate, promote personal responsibility, encourage proactive care, and harness self-interest (as detailed in chapter 2).

Healthcare providers can use social media to help patients become more engaged and can provide them with appropriate education about their conditions and management options. Truly engaged patients who are educated, informed, motivated, inspired, and empowered to work with their healthcare team will ultimately get the best results.

Engaging patients and families improves healthcare outcomes, and it is an important goal of the Electronic Healthcare Records Incentive Program. As the second of five health policy priorities, this policy is designed to improve patients' understanding of their own health and related conditions so they can take a more active role in their own healthcare. It also encourages the involvement of patients' families, as many patients depend on their families for ongoing support.

Engaging patients helps them to be more informed regarding their own medical conditions, and engaged patients are more likely to comply with their providers' recommendations. Well-informed, engaged patients are also better at communicating important health information to their providers, which can assist their providers in making better diagnoses and creating more effective treatment care plans.[23]

Informed and educated patients and their families can take active roles in healthcare decision making. For example, when faced with multiple treatment options, educational materials and tools can help patients more fully participate in their treatment decisions and make better, more informed, personal healthcare choices.

Social media offers new tools for healthcare providers to help their patients make better decisions. As unhealthy lifestyles, habits, and behaviors continue to rise, it is imperative for providers to help patients make better healthy living changes that fit patients' lifestyles. Social media can provide patients with information, education, inspiration, support, mentoring, and accountability.

A positive support system and an accountability program are vital components for a successful healthy living program, and provider-driven social media methodologies offer both the support system and accountability. Not too long ago, there were few, if any, options for healthcare providers to stay in touch with and continue offering support to patients who needed more than quarterly or yearly face-to-face contact. Today, keeping virtually connected with patients is possible and encouraged by pay-for-performance reimbursement.

Goal Setting

Using social media to make personal healthcare goals public is an excellent way for many people to maintain consistency and continue making healthier decisions when they may not feel like it, or when progress slows. Knowing that others are watching can help patients perpetuate successful healthy living habits.[24]

In addition to using social media for goals, patients have many opportunities to connect with fitness experts, medical personnel, and other healthcare providers via their professional pages on Facebook or by following them on Twitter. Many providers enjoy engaging with their patients and answering questions; providing educational content; and suggesting options for meals, workouts, and healthy living tools. Having 24/7 access to so much information can be an incredible tool to promote positive health outcomes.

Improving Patient Healthcare Outcomes

YouTube and Facebook help build relationships, increase engagement, spread information, and keep people entertained. These are not tools providers would immediately think of to promote improved healthcare outcomes or to help patients achieve a healthier lifestyle. Regardless, social media can be a great resource for improving patients' health. Below are five recommendations providers can give to their patients regarding how to use social media to achieve their healthcare goals.

- **Set Goals**—When talking about healthy living, the most difficult requirement is maintaining consistency. It is difficult for patients to regularly go to the gym or make better nutritional choices. Therefore, in order to maintain the necessary consistency, patients must set clear goals for themselves. Healthcare providers should encourage patients to use their personal social media platforms to announce their goals to their friends. Goals should be achievable, objective, and specific and include a date for completion. After announcing their goals, patients need to write a blog, send tweets, and/or post Facebook status updates regarding their progress. This social networking method is a good way for patients to focus on their goals, but it also provides an opportunity for friends, coworkers, and families to offer ongoing feedback, support, and encouragement. Using Google Calendar or another reminder service can also help reinforce patients' abilities to focus on their health goals.

- **Conduct Research**—Once patients set their healthcare goals, they should research the best ways to achieve their goals. The Internet has nearly unlimited information, and doing research can ensure that patients are more aware of their options. YouTube offers thousands of informational videos from health experts. Also, there are blogs and news articles available from quick, easy Internet searches. Healthcare providers should remind patients to use multiple sources, because one information source may not have all the answers. Using multiple sources will reduce the risk of getting misinformation.

- **Use Social Groups**—Healthcare support groups are used by millions of people to share experience, knowledge, motivation, and insight. Providers should tell their patients that they are not alone. No one has to work to get healthy on his or her own, especially when there are peer-to-peer support groups available. Patients need to connect with friends using a Google Group or find new friends on a health social network like Gimme 20 (http://gimme20. com/), Daily Burn (http://dailyburn.com/), or Twit2Fit (https://twitter.com/Twit2Fit) to compare, support, and discuss results.

- **Track Progress**—Providers must encourage patients to maintain up-to-date numbers that represent the progress that has been made. Social networking applications like FitDay (http://www.fitday.com) and iPhone apps like My Weight Loss Coach (http://myweightlosscoachgame.us.ubi.com/) are excellent tools for this.

- **Help Others**—After working hard to meet their personal goals, patients should be encouraged to share their insight, experiences, knowledge, and compassion with others.

Public Health

Due in large part to the Internet and social media, the practice of public health in the United States is rapidly evolving. Until now, the tremendous contributions of public health organizations and professionals have been undervalued by the public. They have been overshadowed by the attention given to institutions and providers who offer direct medical care. However, with the new overarching healthcare industry mandate regarding patient education and prevention, the public health profession is finally getting the recognition it has long deserved.

In the last few years, there has been growing awareness that achieving better community health will require more emphasis on social media–based communication for health promotion and disease prevention. Using social media is an excellent way to aid public health practitioners with educating, informing, mentoring, and inspiring individuals within a community to make healthier living choices that improve their lives.

Even though the United States spends more than any other country on healthcare and has made significant gains in health over time, it ranks poorly on measures of health compared with the rest of the industrialized world. It is clear that destructive behaviors to personal health such as tobacco use, improper nutrition, and lack of physical activity are key causal factors for the nation's decreasing health standards.

Social networking can certainly support existing public health efforts as well as develop new communication methods aimed at improving healthcare outcomes. Social media can be used to monitor the community's health status; design and implement interventions aimed at minimizing health problems; enforce innovative, cutting-edge programs; and evaluate the impact of the interventions.

Social media and social networking strategies can assist public health agencies in the following ways:

- Monitor community health status to identify community health problems.
- Inform, educate, engage, and empower people regarding health issues.
- Develop collaborative social networking–based communities to identify and solve health problems.
- Develop social media strategies that support individual and community health efforts.
- Link people to needed health services and online support communities.
- Evaluate the effectiveness, accessibility, and quality of social media communication to make positive changes.
- Research and use innovative social media–based communication solutions to mitigate health problems.

Using social media for public health purposes will require a change in organizational infrastructure and philosophy. Public health departments can use social media to reach at-risk populations for emerging diseases like HIV/AIDS, SARS, and drug-resistant tuberculosis.

It is a core principle of public health to ensure that current healthcare communication and scientific advances are being utilized.

As public health professionals and organizations better understand and use social media to improve health in the United States, there will be a shift in how communication services are delivered.

Cutting-edge social media development is being used in varied capacities in public health agencies nationwide. Social media public health communication can reach the overwhelming majority of people regardless of race, ethnicity, socioeconomic status, income, location, occupation, housing, religion, or political affiliation. The focus of public health must be to use the most effective communication methodologies to improve the overall health of the population and increase the amount of relevant information available to all groups.

The following are three current healthcare social media examples using hashtags:

1. **#IGotIt4 Flu Campaign**

   Riverdale's Bridgepoint Active Healthcare has launched an interactive social media campaign to encourage people to get the flu shot. The #igotit4 Flu Campaign calls on people to post whom they got the flu shot for on the hospital's social media accounts using the hashtag #igotit4.

2. **#TellCancer**

   Allegheny Health Network (AHN) is focusing a new social media effort to build a community of hope for those affected by cancer. Using the hashtag Tell Cancer (#TellCancer), the network provides a platform for people to send personal messages to cancer. The messages will be gathered and shared via Allegheny Health's social media network and website. The #TellCancer campaign is designed to give people in the community an opportunity to send a message of hope and support that will be shared with others who are facing the same or similar situations.

3. **#IWillListen**

   The campaign is simple: Anyone can make a pledge on Twitter, Facebook, or another social networking platform using the hashtag #IWillListen and any additional commentary they wish to add. The pledge indicates that they are ready to talk and open up to colleagues, friends, and family members living with mental illness, and that they will provide nonjudgmental support. This allows the mentally ill to identify individuals they can talk to, including people who will be safe to disclose mental health issues to, and find friendly ears, support, and help with accessing potentially complex care needs.

Healthcare Apps Improve Patient Health Outcomes

Mobile health apps represent an area of incredible innovation. Patients and their doctors are able to use these apps to obtain, share, and give information quickly and efficiently. These apps can save patients time and money, and some apps can save lives. Healthcare apps connected to wearable devices, for example, are becoming common. Patients diagnosed with chronic high blood pressure can wear a wrist monitor that takes their blood pressure several times a day and transmits the information to a smartphone app. The app then sends the information to the doctor.[34]

Expectant parents now can track their unborn baby's heartbeat with the handheld ultrasound devices pioneered by iCareNewLife. With a smartphone and tablet app, parents can see the baby's heartbeats and share it on their social media pages with family members and friends.

Alzheimer's is one of the leading causes of death in America, but mobile apps are providing a means to collect data and offer treatment to those suffering from the disease, as well as potentially finding a way to prevent it. Several industries are creating recall game apps to stimulate brain activity and prevent or delay the effects of dementia. Some apps have even worked on using facial recognition technology and photo prompts to help patients remember their loved ones.[35]

It's always frustrating to go to the emergency room with a twisted ankle or a fever just to sit for hours waiting to see a doctor. Now, there are mobile apps that provide ER wait times for multiple local facilities. Some hospital emergency rooms have mobile apps that allow online check-in well before a patient arrives, and in some nonlife-threatening cases, the apps can allow a patient to check in, set an appointment time, and wait at home.[36]

Sometimes people have so many prescriptions they can hardly keep track of them all—and that can be deadly. Mobile apps can set reminders for medication dosage and time. They can be used to track medication intake and can notify caregivers if a medication is missed. There are apps that will track allergies and give patients healthy living tips from the convenience of a smartphone. Some health apps give the patient instant mobile medical advice. Pregnancy apps guide women throughout the entire course of their pregnancy, from preconception to postpartum. Diabetes apps can help monitor and record blood sugar levels and send treatment reminders.[37]

The mobile app has enabled more patient-doctor interactions and increased patient and family engagement in an easier and much more cost-effective way. In a vast field with many varying needs, mobile apps are reaching increasing numbers of patients. In addition to social media strategies, mobile healthcare apps will be a critical element to positively impact patient healthcare outcomes.

Patients can use applications to track food, medication, water intake, steps taken, and so on. Tremendous success stories come from people who are accountable to the application and make it public for guidance and support (social media). Patients can reach their goals much more quickly than expected because they use more of the new social media and Internet tools. For instance, they can achieve weight loss using an app to help them drink more water, a website to schedule their workouts, and a comprehensive mobile application to track their food intake.[26]

Eliminating Limiting Factors

Social media eliminates the time and distance factors that many individuals face. It eliminates many cost issues as well, enabling people to get basic guidance for low or no cost. Many companies also offer discounts and incentives to people who are connected to their social media outlets, which enables the patients to gain more complete, detailed information needed to reach personal healthcare goals.

Social media is in no way a replacement for complete programming and personal attention administered by a qualified healthcare professional; however, in this day and age, it certainly makes sense that social media should be an integral part of a provider's support and education system.

Consistency

Consistency will be a key element for creating patient successes in using social media to exceed Meaningful Use Patient and Family Engagement standards. To maximize positive healthcare behavioral changes using social media, there must be consistency in creating and disseminating relevant patient information content. Providers need to clearly define the behaviors they are trying to change and then ensure that the virtual encounters and virtual patient relationships support changing those behaviors. As with a brick-and-mortar practice, there should be consistency in the provider's communications that reflects the organization's written mission, vision, values, and goals.

Consistency is essential for creating a quality experience that can change behavior and improve outcomes. As the healthcare industry adopts more Meaningful Use Patient and Family Engagement standards, and as reimbursement shifts to the pay-for-performance model, consistently using social media tools to create better outcomes will become increasingly important.

Patient Satisfaction

Patient satisfaction has always been a major concern for healthcare providers. Now, with the change in pay-for-performance reimbursement, patient satisfaction will be more important, because this can now impact reimbursement.

More than just reimbursement, patient satisfaction also affects liability risk, customer service, and word-of-mouth marketing. From the liability point of view, patients who are satisfied with their care are less likely to file complaints or lawsuits. From the marketing and customer service point of view, high patient satisfaction levels are crucial to attract new patients, retain existing patients, receive additional word-of-mouth patient referrals, and increase staff morale.

- Healthcare providers should use technology to improve patient satisfaction. Interactive monitors help boost patient satisfaction by 42 percent and increase overall patient satisfaction scores by at least 10 percent.[27]
- Seventy-eight percent of Americans believe doctors who use a computer system to store medical records provide them with better care.[28]

Technology-based solutions can (1) provide staff with information that has been verified and authenticated prior to the patient visit, (2) protect patient confidentiality, and (3) allow patients to communicate with staff and access information about their own care. Using the newest technological tools also increases patient satisfaction and profitability.[28]

Additionally, online patient scheduling systems can provide convenient access to scheduling and refills as well as a platform to respond to questions. E-prescribing programs benefit busy patients as the prescription is sent directly to the pharmacy, eliminating the need for paper prescriptions and allowing patients to pick up their medications faster.

Customer relationship–management tools offer automated e-mail appointment reminders. This tool is helpful to patients, and it reduces the no-show rate for busy healthcare providers. Clinical decision support tools and clinical protocol compliance tracking tools can help providers enhance the care they give to their patients, which will improve patient satisfaction.

Reaching Teens Using Social Media

Communicating health messages with the teenage population has always been a struggle for adolescent healthcare providers. Attempts to get the majority of teens to engage in conversations about their health during an office visit can quickly lead to deafening silence. Most providers are at minimum ten years older than their patients. Thus, it becomes imperative to adopt communication strategies that are relevant to teens. However, many healthcare providers are still resistant to join the digital world.

Social media offers the clinician an opportunity to listen to questions and discover trends in teen health that might not make it to the office. Online platforms allow teen patients to ask anonymous questions in a nonthreatening format. Allowing for patient questions and answers is a good way to supplement conversations in the examination rooms. Social media won't replace conversations between healthcare providers and patients, but giving advice and relevant information online is a better choice for the patients who want more information using other Internet-based communication methods.

As in any social media strategy, effective communication should be adapted to patient demographics. A fourteen-year-old urban teen might have entirely different information needs from a suburban minority teen. Listening to conversations within the specific patient population will help identify the appropriate topics and social media channels that optimize communication to this target audience.[29]

Although online communication may be a smart and convenient way to reach patients, practitioners still need to exercise confidentiality in an ethical and responsible manner. Protecting patient confidentiality is still a priority for clinicians engaging in social media. HIPAA guidelines indicate that digital communication falls under the same standards for protecting patient privacy. Therefore, healthcare providers should never discuss any specific patient cases in online conversations, and they should not accept personal friend requests from patients.

- Bottom of Form

Engaging Baby Boomers

Educating seniors to use Internet tools will be an important part of getting them to better manage their own healthcare and make better choices. Growing numbers of senior citizens are now seeking Internet options for managing their healthcare. Only ten years ago, talking about elderly people using the Internet as a tool to help manage their healthcare would have been inconceivable. However, there are a growing number of Internet-savvy seniors who are using the web to get more information regarding healthcare.[30]

Healthcare providers and accountable care organizations need to include seniors and help them track and virtually manage their care outside of the doctor's office using the Internet. As older people become more comfortable using the Internet, organizations need to consider how newer technologies can make healthcare more accessible and convenient for patients of all ages. To get seniors involved in their own care via the Internet, it is important to teach them how to sign up and use different Internet platforms.

The senior demographic is grossly overlooked on social media. Those sixty-five and older are changing. They are living longer, becoming more active, and growing increasingly literate online. Not only does this age group have forty-seven times the net worth of households headed by those thirty-five and younger (according to *AdAge*), but they are now the fastest growing users of social media. They don't just have an e-mail account; they are searching on Google, browsing Facebook newsfeeds, and watching YouTube, sometimes from their iPads. According to the Pew

Research Center's Internet & American Life Project, there are currently thirty-nine million people aged sixty-five and older using Facebook, Twitter, and Skype, making them the fastest growing age demographic on these sites.

While people are starting to notice more and more grandparents on their Facebook accounts, the figures are actually much greater. According to an All Assisted Living Homes 2010 report, 11 percent of Facebook users are seniors. These 14.8 million users represent a 1,448 percent yearly growth in this demographic. More and more classes are being held to train senior citizens on how to use online tools like Facebook, and 20 percent of these users will log on for an hour on any given day. Pew Research found that 13 percent of adults fifty years and older are already using Twitter and estimate this figure will only continue rising.[79]

Merrill Gardens is one of the leading assisted living centers in America, with more than seven thousand residents and more than fifty communities. The company uses social media to connect with both their residents and the residents' children. In terms of marketing, Merrill Gardens uses social media for lead generation with the adult children of their target market, who are researching homes for their parents online. Beyond lead generation, their Facebook, Twitter, and Instagram accounts are used as a way for residents to stay involved with community events, as well as for adult children to follow the events and news of their parents' assisted living homes. They even have a Pinterest account with creative boards specifically for senior citizens, including "Love at Merrill Gardens," "Top 10 Merrill Gardens Moments," and "Knitting Inspiration."[79]

The American Association of Retired Persons (AARP) is a nonprofit organization providing a wide range of benefits to people aged fifty and older. With more than forty million members, AARP is one of the largest service providers for this age group. According to AARP, the top four online activities for people older than sixty are Google, Facebook, Yahoo, and YouTube, and the organization has tailored its social media similarly. The content on their Twitter, Facebook, and YouTube accounts is targeted directly to their older members, with posts often referring to members' grandchildren or offering tips for staying healthy.

Healthcare Organizations Targeting Senior Citizens

For healthcare providers that target senior citizens but have never considered social media, now is a good time to start. Brands that already have social media strategies might want to consider having separate accounts so the content can be catered to an older demographic. Aside from the type of content, the same principles apply in creating a social media plan: have a focused target, engage with users, listen carefully, and commit to frequent use. Healthcare providers must also narrow their target focus—knowing whether they are targeting senior citizens or their children.

According to *AdAge*, every day for the next two decades, ten thousand boomers will become seniors. At the very least, healthcare providers need to start understanding how to use social media marketing to reach senior citizens.

Connected Living (http://www.connectedliving. com/)

Connected Living is an online community for seniors that is available primarily through senior living centers. The social network was designed to integrate with other tools, such as calendars, menus, and private communications with family members. Users connect with online and real-world friends, and the virtual community allows seniors to see their grandchildren's Instagram photos or share their own photos.

In 2015, people born during the Baby Boom years will be ages fifty to sixty-eight. Using social media to connect with someone in their fifties is very different from connecting with people in their twenties. Baby Boomers are in a different stage of life with different experiences, wants, and needs, so healthcare communication professionals and providers must recognize the need to use different messages and tools to connect with older patients. The following five points include some general information to better understand how to connect with the Baby Boomer generation and virtually improve patient outcomes for older patients. [32]

1. Individuals – Social media content, communication and marketing that invokes social status benefits does not play as well in older markets. Less worried about the reactions of others, older patients lean toward greater practicality in healthcare buying decisions.

2. Intelligent Choices — Older patients are interested in straight facts. Healthcare providers need to give their more mature patients clear, relevant, and valuable information, not a sales pitch.

3. Altruistic—Older patients tend to respond to marketing appeals reflecting altruistic values. As people become older, altruistic motivations become stronger, and narcissistic and materialistic values decrease.

4. Increased Time Making Decisions—Older patients, especially those who are retired, often ignore time-urgency strategies in marketing—such as "buy now".

5. More Complex—Older patients have a decreased sensitivity to price and an increased sensitivity to affordability and value. [33]

Monitoring Results

According to the new healthcare standards, patient and family engagement and interaction will be important for healthcare providers. Engagement expands healthcare provider perspectives; increases positive influence over patients; and secures new, valuable input and interaction. Follower counts, retweets, favorites, likes, and subscribers by themselves have little value to providers who want to change patient outcomes.

Relevant content needs to be provided to engage patients and their families on a personal, emotional, and intellectual level. Shares on social media can be meaningful, but not when they are explicitly demanded as the price of entry for something else. Providers need to pay attention to the interactions that happen organically, not the ones that are manufactured or are being arbitrarily measured by an analytics program.

Likes, shares, and retweets don't show evidence of patient engagement. Social media networks don't know and don't care about the healthcare practice's goals to improve patient outcomes. So why should providers use one of their prepackaged analytics programs to measure success? The best way for providers to measure their social media, goal-oriented performance is to decide on their social media engagement and determine key performance indicators (KPI).

Conclusion

Going forward, healthcare providers will increasingly use social media to virtually connect with their patients. They will also use other technological advances and mobile apps that improve patient outcomes. Although the most likely users of a healthcare engagement program will be tech-savvy young adults, the fifty-plus population must be included as older adults utilize healthcare more frequently. Seniors who have online access and communicate with their physicians help minimize trips to the doctor's office, phone calls, and other interactions that may be more physically challenging, especially if the patient has disabilities or if significant travel distance is involved.

4

Enterprise Social Networking (Internal Communication)

In Web 2.0, Internet-based engagement was the focus of innovative social networking services such as Facebook, YouTube, Twitter, and LinkedIn. The dynamic user interaction of the web quickly became part of everyday life. With the capabilities that social networking services currently offer and with the start of Web 3.0, there are unprecedented opportunities to expand collaboration and information sharing among and between healthcare professionals, employees, departments, specialties, managers, and administrators.

After analyzing more than four thousand companies to see how they used social technologies, McKinsey concluded that the opportunity cost for not using social media is $900 billion to $1.3 trillion yearly. The largest percentage in lost income, 66 percent, was derived from not using social media technologies to initiate better internal communications and collaboration across a business. This study suggests that healthcare businesses can use social media as an internal organizational management tool to increase efficiency, effectiveness, productivity, and profitability.[39]

Internal social networking programs give healthcare organizations the potential to share information, coordinate training, build morale, create teams, and connect employees. Thus, the use of social networking as an internal healthcare organizational communication tool is rapidly expanding. This shift could potentially revolutionize healthcare organizational communication, organizational management, crowdsourced problem solving, staff training, and collaboration.

Internal social networks can play an important role in facilitating collaboration. Some of the most important tasks healthcare professionals perform are locating, using, and disseminating information, and social networking offers effective tools to facilitate these activities. These tools can help professionals with collaborative training, authoring, conferencing, and participating remotely in meetings.

There are many possibilities for collaboration via the Internet. The most popular mainstream technologies include Skype, Google Docs, Twitter, and YouTube. Time-limited healthcare professionals are slowly using new technologies to increase their productivity, but innovation is a process that takes time to incorporate. Additionally, it is difficult, at any point, to propose a single solution for collaboration due to rapid changes in social media development and concurrent changes in a healthcare organization.

There are different categories of social networks, and each category contains a number of social networking sites that, in many cases, are still evolving and expanding but perform similar functions. Each social networking site provides services that address different needs of both the participants and organizations, but the functions available on one site can overlap with another. For instance, the virtual world sites (e.g., Second Life) can provide meeting and collaboration opportunities. Similarly, Facebook (private group) and LinkedIn (private group) can be used to promote research, training, sharing of information, innovation, and collaboration between healthcare professionals as well as healthcare administrators.

Some newer social networking sites such as Google+ provide a large variety of services to promote collaboration, such as Google Hangouts. Any new service proposed by one provider is often replicated in some form by others, with some changes to avoid copyright issues. For example, Circles in Google+ was followed by Groups in LinkedIn, Networks on Ryze, and Lists on Facebook.[39]

Collaboration can include the following information-sharing and engagement classifications:
- Enterprise healthcare software tools.
- Current healthcare information social networks (LinkedIn Groups).
- Databases and platforms.
- Collaborative writing, file sharing, and online storage (Google Docs).
- Conversation, communication, webinars, and video conferencing.
- Presentation-sharing tools (Prezi.com).
- Project management, scheduling, and collaboration tools.

Often the focus is on new technologies, yet the use of existing technologies in different ways can solve problems, increase morale, advance training, maximize communication, and improve organizational effectiveness. Using social media to increase organizational efficiencies doesn't have to be dramatic, awe-inspiring processes.

The shift to internal social networking starts with changing how problems are perceived and modifying existing social media tools to address them. Using social media internally, rather than just as a marketing methodology, is a paradigm shift that will allow healthcare organizations to use platforms that already exist in new, internally productive, and innovative ways.

Internal Social Networking
Using internal social networking within the healthcare sector is a relatively new concept with nearly unlimited possibilities. It

can improve organizational efficiencies and increase profits. For many healthcare organizations, it would be worth the time to make the shift. There are many possible tools to use, including the following more popular platforms: Facebook, Facebook private groups, LinkedIn private groups, blogs, videos, podcasts, Twitter, Pinterest, Instagram, Google+, Google Hangouts, Second Life, webinars, weblogs, Ning, and Spruz.

There are many additional social networking tools for healthcare professionals. The following is a partial list:

1. All Nurses (http://allnurses.com/)—Nurses share photos, stories, and patient questions (along with debates, news, reviews, and other information of interest) with their peers on AllNurses.com. The site has more than 840,000 members, and conversations commonly follow a thread format. The "Nurses Breakroom" area covers general topics, entertainment, and other healthcare and non-healthcare subjects.

2. Doctors Hangout (http://www.doctorshangout.com/)—Doctors Hangout looks a lot like Facebook but features questions about abnormal rashes and estimating insulin doses. It boasts members from around the world, including doctors, medical students, and representatives of professional organizations and medical publications.

3. Ozmosis (http://ozmosis.org/)—Created and supported by enterprise collaboration software developer Ozmosis, this social network is free to all licensed US physicians as a place to share medical knowledge. Ozmosis.org aggregates these data and shares insights about clinical, management, and healthcare practices.

4. QuantiaMD (https://secure.quantiamd.com/)—Similar to a support group, QuantiaMD lets healthcare professionals communicate privately in secure discussions with other members, all identified by name. With a base of approximately two hundred thousand members, QuantiaMD's free site helps physicians with topics such as doctors'

well-being, policy and reform, practice profitability, career development, and more.

5. Sermo (https://www.sermo.com/)—Sermo is designed exclusively for physicians. It provides its more than 270,000 members with clinical tools and resources. Doctors collaborate on patient cases and other medical topics to improve healthcare delivery and patient outcomes. Physicians on Sermo can discuss a topic in an open, supportive environment. They also can participate in market research studies for honoraria; Sermo pays more than $20 million in honoraria to doctors annually.

6. Therapy Networking (http://www.therapynetworking. com/)—The goal of this free social networking community is to create a fun, informative gathering place for therapists, psychologists, marriage counselors, social workers, and psychiatrists to connect, share stories, get support, and make new friends and colleagues. Providers learn how to attract new clients and receive valuable marketing strategy information from experts and therapists who are getting results in their own practices.

Physician Networking

A growing number of doctors are using web-based tools to engage and learn from their colleagues. No matter if it's Doximity (a network that claims three hundred thousand users), Sermo (claiming 270,000 users), or QuantiaMD (claiming 225,000 users), more than ever, physicians are connecting with other physicians.

Improving Internal Communications

Social networking can improve internal communications in four key areas: (1) enhancing collegiality, teamwork, and mutual respect; (2) creating collaboration through transparency; (3) exploiting internal expertise; and (4) perpetuating cross-department training and problem solving.

Within even the smallest healthcare organizations, there are different departments, various levels of training and responsibility, and a diverse employee mix. Getting these components to work together in a team environment is very difficult. For many healthcare companies, social networks can help in this process.

Collegiality, Teamwork, Mutual Respect

Creating an internal healthcare social network will improve communication that leads to collegiality, teamwork, and mutual respect. One of the biggest problems for many healthcare organizations is finding ways to maximize communication between highly diversified groups. Ultimately, lack of effective communication can lead to a significant waste of resources and cost companies millions of dollars. Internal social networks can help people from different parts of the organization develop better communication-based relationships.

When developing internal social networks, healthcare leaders must encourage employees to share posts related to things they are interested in, like photos of their children or grandchildren, vacation pictures, recipes, and life events such as a marriage, birth, or purchase of a new home. Employees who get to know one another's interests and life outside the office will break through some of the petty issues that plague many organizations.

Finding non-work-related common interests can create a sense of community. People who like one another as human beings are more likely to communicate effectively when there is a controversial issue that needs to be discussed and resolved.

Social networking can help create relationships at all levels of an organization, and the leadership needs to be part of the sharing process as well. Leaders need to show their employees that they are "real" human beings, not just their bosses or members of the executive staff. One can imagine the power of team development and morale enhancement when employees learn that the CEO runs marathons on weekends to help raise money for breast cancer awareness, or that the CFO has a daughter the same age, or that the CIO volunteers in a hospice.

Getting employees to share what happens outside of work helps them to connect around areas of common interest. If the only purpose for an internal social network is to provide a forum for employees to share personal experiences, it will still help break down barriers, increase communication, and build morale. If, however, the internal social network is simply a broadcast channel to communicate business information, the networking program will be less effective. For internal social media programs to be effective, organizations have to use the power of *social* in social media to make positive changes and increase communication. The internal social network is an opportunity to build connectivity by engaging employees at all levels and locations.[41]

Collaboration through Transparency

An ongoing challenge is coordinating work and communicating information involving current projects. In many cases, employees keep information to themselves in a protective, proprietary, secretive manner rather than sharing it. Promoting an open communication environment to share information has several benefits. First, it is possible that others may be working on or know something that could benefit an ongoing project. Second, the project may overlap with other employees or departments, and a larger plan for coordinating activities could improve the overall success of the project.

Employees or groups often focus on a project that could turn into something more significant if they combined forces with other employees to solve the greater organizational problem. Healthcare organizations need to use social networking to create opportunities where employees share information on current projects and post status updates on their progress.

To maximize inter-organizational collaboration, employees should be given opportunities to do the following: (1) create cross-functional teams for projects, (2) invite collaborators, (3) subscribe to receive updates, (4) ask to join a project team, (5) list the types of projects that could impact their jobs or departments, and (6) provide a list of requested updates. If healthcare organizations can use a social network for information sharing and collaboration around the actual work performed, they can create tremendous efficiencies for the entire organization.

Exploit Internal Expertise

Healthcare organizations need to provide a searchable database where employees can list their professional experience and talents. Too often, organizations have no idea that needed expertise is available in-house, and they ultimately hire high-priced consultants to do jobs that current employees can do.

Along with professional experience and talent, the internal employee database should include information about employees' outside interests. When a group has a project, they might be able to find a current employee who could add to the project's success. For instance, if an employee is passionate about photography and studied it in his free time, that employee could be the photographer at the next business-sponsored event. The employee would, most likely, be excited about working on a project involving something he is passionate about, and the company could identify talent that could save money and time.

Internal Improvement Ideas Using Social Media

Physicians, nurses, and staff can participate in a social media–style voting system to produce a set of principles for improving care. The crowdsourced program would allow all staff to anonymously suggest ideas on how services can be made more integrated, patient centered, and efficient. Using an innovative platform, support staff would be able to vote "thumbs up" or "thumbs down" if they agree with the proposed ideas. This simple use of internal social media would unlock the expertise and creativity that is currently untapped within the workforce.

Tapping Untapped Talent
Every healthcare business has potential opportunities that it doesn't have the time and resources to pursue. Additionally, nearly every healthcare business has a wealth of internal employee talent and knowledge that goes unused. Using social networking, employees could propose projects they want to work on and list the talents they could bring to a cross-functional team.

Employee-driven social networking could transform how opportunities are researched and pursued. Instead of the traditional approach of requiring an executive to lead the internal innovation, this democratic social networking environment would recognize the value of employees as potential innovators.

Kaiser Permanente's IdeaBook[42]
IdeaBook is Kaiser Permanente's internal social media collaboration platform that supports blogs, wikis, and chats. It supports virtual groups and cross-functional virtual work teams. IdeaBook is where employees are able to have conversations behind a secure firewall about how business is done within the organization.

IdeaBook also supports videos and allows employees to both share them internally and embed them in an intranet page. Internal video sharing has been very valuable for Kaiser to ensure that all internal videos don't end up on YouTube.

Having the ability to share video information has proven to be an important aspect of IdeaBook. A healthcare department manager, for instance, could request that each of her ten employees comes up with solutions to a well-defined departmental problem. Then, the solutions would be posted on an intranet group page where other team members could comment on them. This process would allow all the people in the department to collaborate online in a secure space where they can freely share information without losing it in e-mails, offline conversations, or offline documents.

The compelling value of using a secure intranet comes from creating groups across the organization that wouldn't otherwise exist. Employees who use an intranet are engaging in conversations in their areas of expertise. They can also engage in conversations that are outside their areas of expertise but are well within their areas of interest and curiosity. Using a confidential internal social media communication tool can be very valuable for promoting collaboration in a safe, effective, internal communication environment.

It is, of course, not easy for healthcare organizations to handle all the privacy concerns about confidential information when opening up public forums to employees. For example, Kaiser Permanente's internal social media IdeaBook is governed by a document called the Principles of Responsibility. These principles are very clear about addressing privacy concerns and confidential information. Member data must remain absolutely private, and every employee is trained to respect confidential information both in online and offline environments.[43]

Social Media Business Applications

Healthcare human resource departments are using social media (LinkedIn, etc.) to find, connect, and recruit job seekers and streamline the application process. Sales teams use social media to generate leads and track clients. Operations and distribution teams forecast supply chains, while research and development groups brainstorm product ideas using online virtual meeting platforms. The idea that social media is solely a marketing tool is shifting to its acceptance as a serious business tool.

E-mail as an internal business communication tool has remained essentially unchanged since the first networked message was sent in 1971. To this day, e-mail continues to be an excellent one-to-one, formal correspondence method. However, there are far better tools for internal healthcare organization collaboration. In fact, instant messaging, wikis, Google Drive, and cloud-based computing are becoming an integral part of healthcare organizational employee interactions that allows for real-time communication and centralized information sharing.

Increasingly powerful internal healthcare communication tools are available or in development. Many of these tools use features available on popular networks like Facebook. In 2015 internal business networks like Yammer and Chatter will increase in healthcare organization popularity. These enterprise social networks enable employees to form virtual work groups and exchange ideas on centralized message boards. Among the greatest value of these tools is their ability to make previously little-known information more transparent and make relevant content accessible and searchable for the entire organization.

Big Data
Social media has given healthcare organizations access to unprecedented amounts of information on patient behavior and preferences (i.e., Big Data). However, making sense of so much information and turning it into an actionable policy has been difficult. Larger organizations like Dell, Gatorade, and the Red Cross have led the way by creating dedicated command centers for real-time monitoring and analysis. In 2015 the technology used in complex command centers will likely be compressed on single monitors or even smartphone screens. At a glance, healthcare executives and department managers can see real-time analysis of social metrics and use this information to make better, more informed, real-time, internal business decisions.[43]

Conclusion
In 2005, Mayo Clinic, a pioneer in using healthcare social media, began a journey to improve healthcare globally, using social media methodologies. They formed the Mayo Clinic Center for Social Media. The Mayo Clinic uses internal social networking tools like Yammer to help organize conversations, reduce email clutter, and

keep documents all together so everyone involved can participate and track progress.

Internal healthcare enterprise social networking is flattening organizations by distributing access to key information across all levels within the organization. Additionally, new internal social networking tools continue to be introduced and used. The opportunities for healthcare organizations, from hospitals to single provider offices, are enormous. The growing use of electronic health records, the explosion of mobile device use among healthcare providers, and the rise of the social enterprise give healthcare staff and clinical professionals instant access to information.[44]

5

SOCIAL MEDIA STRATEGY
(Getting Started)

MANY HEALTHCARE ORGANIZATIONS have Facebook fan pages, but what was the purpose of starting these pages? How does a Facebook fan page fit into an overall business organizational development plan? How does a Facebook page help to increase an organization's success? How is the time working on a page being monitored regarding the return on investment, and/or is there a lost opportunity for not doing something other than Facebook that would get better results?

Simply having a Facebook and/or Twitter page does not make a healthcare organization social media savvy. Understanding how target audiences interact with and are influenced by social media is complex. Before starting to use social media and joining the conversation, it is important to listen and monitor what is currently being communicated in social media about the organization. A healthcare organization must listen first to better understand where to focus its communication resources and to determine what messages would best support the organizational goals and objectives.

Seven Social Media Tools Healthcare Providers Should Consider Using

Healthcare providers can no longer rely on their patients to recommend them to friends and family. An online presence is not just recommended but it is now required.

1. LinkedIn—Healthcare providers should not limit their LinkedIn interactions to only building their list of professional contacts. Instead, a provider should create a company page that opens another line of communication for patients.

2. Facebook—Facebook is a social media giant. It offers a simple platform that can be used to share public information. By consistently sharing on the site, healthcare providers can keep their names on the forefront of their current patients' minds while increasing their exposure to potential new patients.

3. Yellow Pages—Yellow Pages no longer arrive as a book. Instead, the brand has reinvented itself as an online search engine for businesses. Doctors should take advantage of this and list their practices here. This is also a tool that does not need to be used extensively. Healthcare providers can set plans to check their profiles once every month and make note of any reviews left.

4. Yelp—Similar to Yellow Pages which hosts business profiles, Yelp varies as it is used heavily by individuals looking to read reviews and ratings on a particular healthcare provider. Providers should make profiles and monitor reviews posted on Yelp more consistently (Yelp is updated more frequently than other rating sites). If there is a negative review, a provider can improve his/her practice or respond to the patient directly online to resolve the issue.

5. Angie's List—While Yelp and Yellow Pages are open to the public, Angie's List is a subscription-based site that offers reviews that hold a little more weight than those

posted on free sites. Creating a profile is free, which allows healthcare providers an opportunity to increase their exposure.

6. Twitter—Twitter allows healthcare providers to share their personalities in a professional setting. Some ideas to tweet about could include health-related inspirational quotes or breaking news in the healthcare industry.

7. YouTube—Healthcare professionals can share brief, medically focused videos to inform patients.

Questions to ask when developing a healthcare social media campaign:

- What are the organization's mission, vision, goals, and objectives?
- Specifically, which target groups could benefit the organization?
- Which social media channels would help the organization to be more successful? Internal? External? Both?
- Which resources should be allocated to create and maintain these new social media channels of communication?
- What positive impacts or results can be expected from ongoing conversations on multiple specifically selected platforms with various target groups?

It is vital for every healthcare organization to listen to what patients and target groups who are active in social media are saying. Having a better understanding and analyzing what is happening on the Internet can be done with listening data-mining platforms like Nuvi (http://www.nuvi.com/) and Radian6 (http://www.salesforcemarketingcloud.com/).

Healthcare organizations have always had the ability to survey key publics. Now, with the Internet, organizations large and small have access to a much larger data set to gain insight that can be used for improving and developing new and existing programs, products, and services; improving customer-relationship management services; completing an ongoing competitive analysis; and predicting future needs.

Creating and managing social media have the potential to utilize a significant amount of resources with little real results. For social media to be effective, a plan needs to be written to manage the organization's social media efforts over time. Writing a comprehensive social media strategy is the only rational response to ensure that all internal parties are working toward the same goals. The plan can determine what platforms should be used, what resources should be made available, and what results should be expected.

Creating a social media strategy with defined goals is the only way to ensure that using this form of communication will generate a return on investment. Additionally, a social media strategy is needed because social media is always changing. The way social media works overall and the functionality within each platform are always in flux.

With so many changes in social media, the strategies used yesterday may not be as effective today, and will most certainly be out of date tomorrow. Furthermore, a one-time strategy without review and alterations may limit the use of new, emerging networking opportunities. In other words, a social media strategy can help healthcare organizations focus their efforts, optimize the results, and respond to future changes as they occur, but they must be very flexible to adapt to a quickly changing technology environment.

When using social media, what are the goals the organization is trying to achieve? Social media business objectives and projected outcomes require clearly defined goals. Start with the current business strategy, and look at the key points to see where social media could help to achieve, accelerate, or enhance the organization's potential for success.

The following are examples of how healthcare organizations can use social media:

1. **Increase Income**
   - Increase brand awareness.
   - Start and promote a new product or service.
   - Improve patient retention rate and increase sales.
   - Develop new business.

- Increase word-of-mouth referrals.
- Generate more Internet traffic to a website or physical location.
- Use social media, especially with e-commerce, as the primary marketing method.

2. **Improve Customer-Relationship Management**
   - Respond to negative feedback.
   - Use negative feedback to improve services and products.
   - Engage key groups in ongoing conversations.
   - Survey key publics regarding their needs and wants.
   - Respond to positive comments.
   - Disseminate valuable, relevant information.
   - Stay in contact with key publics.
   - Inform key publics about new products and services.
   - Inform key publics about any changes within the organization and/or industry.
   - Expand the organizational brand to improve public goodwill.

3. **Decrease Expenses**
   - Reduce the need to use recruiting agencies for new employees and clinical staff.
   - Shift some of the traditional marketing budget to social media to see if a better return on investment can be achieved at a reduced cost.

4. **Improve Patient Healthcare Outcomes**
   - Virtually engage existing patients to provide information, inspiration, monitoring, and education.
   - Provide accurate, relevant health information.
   - Provide opportunities for patients to support one another.

5. **Improve Internal Management**
   - Create a team and minimize proprietary behavior.
   - Increase morale.
   - Improve collaboration.
   - Enhance internal communication.

- Promote employee participation, feedback, and employee-initiated organizational improvement programs.
- Increase training options.
- Improve and increase information sharing within specialties.
- Impact the success rate of developing programs.

6. **Control Organizational Social Media**
- Train every employee regarding the use of social media (personal and work related).
- Train every employee on how to maintain patient privacy and patient confidentiality.
- Write internal social media policies and procedures that include patient confidentiality; government affairs; mutual respect; political activity; employee computer, e-mail, and Internet use; and photography, video, and release of patient information.
- Establish an infrastructure to monitor, support, and govern internal social media efforts.

7. **Become More Informed**
- Get real-time information (Twitter, etc.).
- Participate in groups that have leaders and innovators in your sector.
- Use RSS feeds to get information as it is disseminated.

Branding

To create a comprehensive social media strategy, certain elements need to be in the plan, and although there is some overlap, elements should be listed individually to provide more clarity. Social media development within a healthcare organization must also be consistent. The name, logo, color scheme, and voice all need to be the same.

Name—Every account in social media should have the same name as your company. If there is extra room in the name area, add keywords to increase search engine optimization. At the beginning, all social media platforms should be similar, singular in focus, and representative of the entire business.

Color Scheme—The color scheme for a brand's social media presence should already be clearly spelled out in the company's brand guidelines. Social media needs to adhere to these.

Voice—The voice in social media is equivalent to the tone of its conversations. Traditional communication standards would be more appropriate for written correspondence, but in social media the organizational voice is expected to be more conversational. Also, healthcare is about people and relationships. So it is important to modify the tone so that it is easily accepted by a broad range of participants with whom the organization is attempting to complete an ongoing dialogue.

Content

When executing a social media strategic plan, there is some content sharing between platforms. Sharing relevant content helps cultivate brand awareness and trust. A healthcare organization's news, as well as content acquired from other sources that the targeted demographic would deem valuable, should be shared through social media channels. Although social media is not about self-promoting, the followers of the brand might appreciate this type of message, and in doing so self-promotion can be included on a limited basis.

When sharing self-promotion, especially the automated kind, companies should keep it to a bare minimum. It is important to share content that the organization's customers and potential customers would be interested in receiving. Sharing relevant information in a meaningful and engaging way helps organizations by (1) establishing credibility and goodwill, (2) engendering trust in the brand, (3) building brand awareness, (4) increasing website traffic, and (5) promoting dialogue with targeted social media users that strengthens relationships and builds a stronger, more loyal online community.

The types of content to share in social media formats vary dramatically among different healthcare organizations. The content strategy includes the following: (1) new product or service information; (2) new events, coming events, and highlights from recent events; (3) original blog posts that are targeted articles based on a keyword strategy; (4) YouTube videos added to the organizational channel; (5) photos of products, locations, staff and/or events; (6) conversations from other social media channels such as responses to questions or surveys; (7) engagement questions or quotes (especially for Facebook); (8) content from key publics like guest blog posts, photos, articles, and videos; and (9) third-party information relevant to the target group.

Sharing third-party information allows an organization to serve as a valuable resource. This should be shared in a strategic combination with original content, content from other industry leaders, and content generated by patients and other key publics.

Content Posting

Content posting is an important part of implementing a social media strategy. It includes collecting, organizing, and displaying information relevant to a particular topic or area of interest. This process also lets organizations be viewed less like marketers and more like integrated community resources. Relevant content often comes from news sources and bloggers. For some companies, posting photos from patients and staff can also provide great content.

Here are some ways organizations can find third-party website content to share on their social media channels: (1) using relevant content the staff reads every day that the target group might find interesting; (2) using relevant keywords in Twitter search engines like Topsy.com to see which news or blogs are being frequently retweeted; and (3) creating an RSS reader that secures content from blogs and continuing to add, delete, and modify RSS subscriptions to optimize the content. Note: Organizations should consult with a legal advisor before publishing third-party content.

Channels

Social media has many communities, also referred to as channels. Selecting the right channels in which to participate will have a major impact on the success of an organization's social media strategic plan. A company should use publicly available data found in keyword searches, reading research, and other documentation highlighting demographic information to ensure that the social media channel it is considering is the most appropriate one to help the healthcare business gain success. Although a healthcare organization can participate in an unlimited number of channels, it is strongly recommended that the initial social media campaign start with three or fewer; make them successful before moving on to conquer new ones.

Frequency

For a healthcare business with finite resources, it is important to set guidelines as to the frequency in which content is published on each platform. More frequent blogs and YouTube videos can create more opportunities to be indexed by Google, and therefore more opportunities to appear in search results.

It is recommended that healthcare organizations conservatively post one or two times per week on LinkedIn's and Facebook's business pages. Google+ and Twitter require more frequent posts to be found and heard above the noise. A good goal would be to, at minimum, post twice as much on Twitter and Google+ as is done on LinkedIn and Facebook. Different platforms will require different frequency strategies.

Engagement

To develop a healthcare organization's social media strategy, there are two distinct parts. First there is proactive posting of both new content and conversations, as well as the sharing of information and content from others. Second, there are reactive conversations with social media users, responding to those who comment or message.

Campaign

Using a well defined content strategy and appropriate channels, healthcare social media campaigns are essential to continually engage key publics and attract new ones. For this reason, organizations should use a wide variety of content topics, content types, and channels to increase fan engagement and grow the user base. If it is used externally, internally, or as a tool to help improve patient outcomes, social media should leverage and promote the social aspect of the communication medium.

Crisis Management

Crisis management is covered more in detail in chapter 6. However, it is important to include a thorough crisis management section in the social media strategy. If an organization already has a crisis communications strategy, it is a good idea to plan how to integrate social media with it.

Once a social media strategy is written, it is important to continually review the value and results derived from the different platforms. Then the written strategy should be changed as needed to improve results. A social media strategy plan is not static; it is one moment in time that constantly changes as new information is received.

6

AVOIDING THE OBSTACLES

CHANGING TECHNOLOGIES ARE creating new legal obstacles for healthcare professionals. Out of the chaos created by change, there remains a confusing array of local, regional, national, and international regulatory issues. This chapter is restricted to general guidelines regarding privacy, confidentiality, and the security of information on the Internet.

Technologies continue to expand and evolve exponentially. The regulatory agencies, Internet attorney specialists, and courts are trying their best, but the speed and scope of change make it nearly impossible to stay current. This chapter should not be considered legal advice. If healthcare providers have specific legal questions, they should consult a competent attorney regarding use of the Internet, follow a blog written by an Internet healthcare attorney, and/or follow authority sites to get the newest regulatory information (i.e., FDA.gov, etc.).

The healthcare industry is the subject of many legal actions, so it is difficult for its leaders to move forward without worrying about liability and the possibility of litigation. To avoid obstacles using Internet communication, healthcare organizations should do the following: (1) set up flexible written guidelines, (2) have the guidelines reviewed by a competent attorney who is knowledgeable about the Internet, (3) train every employee, (4) monitor the use of social media, (5) and, most importantly, use common sense.

Social Media Used for the "Right" Reasons

Many healthcare providers and organizations opt out of using social media because of privacy concerns. Many older professionals are new to social media, and they don't understand it or how it can be important. But even though there are risks, there are many more opportunities for using social media. With the addition of written policies, caution, and common sense, social media can enhance the lives of millions of Americans and significantly increase profits for organizations of all sizes. In spite of privacy fears, litigation concerns, and lack of knowledge at the highest levels, social media can and should be used because it is in the best interest of the healthcare organization and the patients it serves.

Having an online presence has its advantages when it comes to healthcare marketing, but it does come with some risks. Patients can share their experiences online with the click of a mouse, and their comments travel quickly through their social networks. Journalists, ever ready for a news scoop, may pick up on the story and run with it. A crisis can then escalate rapidly, and organizations need to be ready to remedy the situation without delay. The only way to do this is to have a crisis plan already in place.

Crisis Management

Crisis management involves dealing with threats before, during, and after they have occurred. Healthcare companies should proactively prepare by developing a crisis response plan and including the following elements:

1. **Define What Constitutes a Crisis**

   Three elements are common to a crisis: (1) a threat to the organization, (2) the element of surprise, and (3) a short decision time. A crisis can fall into several categories including (1) technological (e.g., the company's website has been hacked), (2) confrontation (disgruntled employee, client, or patient attacks the organization online), (3) rumors (e.g., spreading false information about the company online), and (4) malevolence (e.g., in 1982 cyanide was added to Tylenol capsules on store shelves, killing seven people).

2. **Crisis Management Listening**

An effective social media strategy requires active listening to the online chatter about an organization. Should a crisis occur, listening to the conversation will help the company shape a more insightful and effective response. Responding in real time to issues strengthens public perception that the organization's focus is firmly on patient satisfaction. In addition, companies should use monitoring to find the conversations to which they can add value. Investing in community building online will pay dividends in the form of support should a crisis arise.

3. **Crisis Management Written Plan**

   The plan should include the following: (1) clear guidelines on how to respond to each of the different situations; (2) a clear chain of command and list of contact information; and (3) team-wide knowledge about the plan, how to access it, and how to put it into action.

4. **Crisis Management Taking Action**

   The following are key steps and considerations for crisis management healthcare organizations should keep in mind:

   a. Determine the exact nature of the crisis. How is it affecting the company's patients or business?

   b. Go to the source. Find where the complaint originated and with whom. If someone published something that is untrue or misrepresentative, ask them to remove, amend, or modify it if appropriate to do so.

   c. Be respectful, polite, and engaged. Never get into a public disagreement.

   d. Acknowledge the situation and that it is being dealt with.

   e. Respond swiftly and appropriately. Every

moment counts on social media. The longer the organization waits, the more the conversation will heat up. Twitter, in particular, is a platform where people expect a quick response no matter what time of day.

f. Don't lie or try to hide the truth; providers must admit when they are at fault.

Privacy, Confidentiality, and Data Protection

Privacy, confidentiality, and data protection are important concerns when using social media. Professionals should be aware of the implications of the wide range of privacy issues that involve healthcare-related social media so they can respond appropriately to their patients' concerns and needs.

Privacy

In general, privacy is the right to be free from secret surveillance and to determine whether, when, how, and to whom one's personal or organizational information may be revealed.[45]

Confidentiality

This is the entrusting of proprietary information from one party to another for that party's exclusive use so as not to impart the obtained knowledge to others.[46] A patient's informed consent can authorize relaxation of confidentiality for specific information. However, it is important to follow all of the HIPAA regulations related to patient privacy and confidential issues.

Data Protection

Data protection is the process of safeguarding important information from corruption or loss. The term *data protection* is used to describe both operational backup of data and disaster recovery/business continuity (DR/BC).[47]

Professionals have an obligation to protect patient privacy and confidentiality, which also includes the need to ensure adequate security provisions regarding the Internet service provider, website host, website developer, local network, and personal staff computers. All software used in healthcare settings, including social media, should be tested in order to remove predictable situations that can cause a potential breach in protecting patient confidentiality.

Maintaining Patient Trust

The entire healthcare industry depends on eliciting, maintaining, and deserving trust. Patients are often suspicious of material presented via the Internet, so before using an Internet-based platform, it is important to read and understand its privacy policy to better protect patients' privacy and maintain their trust. Many patients fear that disclosure of their medical information could cause irreparable harm to their relationships with family, friends, acquaintances, and business associates.[48] Therefore, healthcare professionals must remain steadfast guardians of patients' confidentiality and privacy.

Health Insurance Portability and Accountability Act

The Office for Civil Rights enforces the HIPAA Privacy Rule, which protects the privacy of individually identifiable health information; the HIPAA Security Rule, which sets national standards for the security of electronic protected health information; the HIPAA Breach Notification Rule, which requires covered entities and business associates to provide notification following a breach of unsecured protected health information; and the confidentiality provisions of the Patient Safety Rule, which protect identifiable information being used to analyze patient safety events and improve patient safety.[49]

Federal regulations have been written by the US Department of Health and Human Services to guarantee to patients new rights and protections against the misuse of disclosure of their health records by providers who transmit health information in electronic form. Patient privacy and confidentiality can also be covered by state regulations. HIPAA has many rules that need to be applied when using social media. However, a full discussion of HIPAA is beyond the expertise and scope of this chapter.

Sharing information on the Internet is becoming the norm, but a seemingly innocent post could be a breach of a patient's privacy and trust. In a society saturated with social media, it is important in healthcare to look not only at the letter of the law, but also the greater meaning or intent. When posting on the Internet, healthcare professionals must consider how the information may be perceived by others.

An Ounce of Prevention

Facebook and other personal social networking sites give healthcare professionals an opportunity to vent online with family and friends after a long, stressful day. It is important for professionals to protect patients' privacy even when they believe they are speaking to a few of their close friends. When using the Internet, information intended for one person, but that should have been kept private, can unintentionally be disseminated to thousands or millions of other listeners, readers, and posters. It is very important for professionals to remember that even in the privacy of their own homes, HIPAA and many state privacy laws prohibit healthcare professionals from disclosing patient information without proper patient authorization.

When professionals use their personal social media pages, they should not post any information, no matter how seemingly harmless, without the patient's consent. HIPAA and many state privacy laws prohibit disclosing patient information regardless if it is during work or after work. Even a shocking picture may violate these laws and lead to fines and other penalties. Additionally, lawsuits or news stories regarding the breach of confidential information through social media can tarnish a provider's reputation.[51]

Often professionals believe they have omitted any identifying patient information in their posts, but clinical details alone could be enough to violate HIPAA. As a good rule to follow, professionals should not use social media to share any health information that could be linked to a patient.[51]

Individually identifiable health information refers to health information that could be used to identify a person. When using social media, avoid any possibility that a patient could be identified. The following is a short list[51] of information that should not be disclosed when using social media:

- A patient's, relative's, or employer's name; address; phone; fax; e-mail address; or geographic information.
- Dates of hospitalization, dates of birth, photographs, or video recordings.
- Social security numbers, medical record numbers, memberships, license numbers, account numbers.
- Health plan beneficiary numbers, and certificate or license numbers.
- Vehicle identifiers and serial numbers, including license plate numbers.
- Device identifiers and serial numbers, URLs, or IP address numbers.
- Biometric identifiers (e.g., finger and voice prints).
- Any other unique identifying numbers, characteristics, or codes.

With the potential risks, it is crucial to take an ounce-of-prevention approach to ensuring employees, contractors, and agents aren't violating patient privacy laws when using social media. This can be done through the creation and implementation of a comprehensive written social media policy. This policy should clearly spell out the expectations of employees' uses of social media, especially when they have the slightest relationship to patient care.[52]

Let employees know the consequences for policy violations before they post to a social networking site. Encouraging staff to report those who violate the policy will increase the organization's ability to monitor, even if passively, the social media activity of their employees. Having a clear policy that is frequently reviewed with staff allows institutions and employers to actively manage risk associated with HIPAA and privacy law violations, as well as prevent the bad press and costs associated with a lawsuit for privacy violations.[52]

Three Commonsense Online Rules

1. Regarding healthcare information and staying in compliance with HIPAA: "If you wouldn't say it offline, don't say it online!" Healthcare professionals must always use their best judgment in social media communications.

2. Professionals must consider that everything they post on the Internet is public and that there is no longer a clear boundary between work life and personal life.

3. Professionals must also remember that the advancement of public health prevails over all other purposes. Regardless of the online source used to communicate, public health is best served by clear, accurate, truthful, and non-misleading information.

Food and Drug Administration (FDA)

Due in large part to US Food and Drug Administration (FDA) oversight, social media raises issues and concerns for people in the healthcare industry. Social media has made information about medical conditions and treatment options quicker and easier to find, and this information often goes beyond what is on a drug label. Unfortunately, social media's content, primarily created by users, may not be accurate.

The FDA protects the public health and recently provided acceptable promotion of regulated product guidelines for public relation firms that use social media and the Internet. These guidelines include how to present risk vs. benefit information on microblogging platforms such as Twitter. The FDA also provided information on how drug and device companies can counter misinformation spread by critics or other users on sites such as Google+, Twitter, Facebook, and Wikipedia.

Staying away from or ignoring social media is not the answer. Instead, getting in the conversation and providing accurate information can improve people's health by giving them the best resources to make better healthcare choices. Always remember that professionals who use social media can improve lives. In addition, they can create organizational efficiencies and increase profits.

Whether the FDA can appropriately regulate a quickly changing social media environment is up for debate. Regardless, it is important to adhere to the FDA's new guidelines as they are developed. People are actively using social media to obtain and share health information. To stay in compliance, healthcare providers should stay consistent with the FDA's newest position on social media; follow the guidelines; and, of course, use common sense.

FDA Draft Guidance on Social Media and Internet Communications

Ongoing changes in technology transform medical products and the ways that both patients and healthcare providers learn about those products. In today's world, in addition to traditional sources of medical product information, patients and healthcare providers regularly get information about FDA regulated medical products through social media and other Internet sources, and those technologies continue to evolve. But regardless of the Internet source used to communicate about medical products, public health is best served by clear, accurate, truthful, and non-misleading information about them. That's why the agency has proposed two draft guidances to ensure that the information provided by drug and device companies is accurate and will help patients to make well informed decisions in consultation with their healthcare providers.

FDA Guidances

The first June 2014 FDA guidance provides recommendations for presenting risk and benefit information for prescription drugs or medical devices using Internet/social media sources with character space limitations, such as Twitter, and the paid search results links on Google and Yahoo.[53] These recommendations address the presentation of both benefit information and risk information in this setting. It is understood that communicating on Internet sites with character space limitations can be challenging. But no matter the Internet source used, benefit claims in product promotions should be balanced with risk information. Companies should provide a way for consumers to gain direct access to a more complete discussion of risks associated with their products.

The FDA June 2014 second guidance provides recommendations to companies that choose to correct third-party information related to their own prescription drugs and medical devices.[54] This draft guidance provides the FDA's recommendations on the correction of misinformation from independent third parties on the Internet and through social media sites.

These new guidances, in part, were developed to respond to requests for best practices from companies and other stakeholders. Prescription drugs and medical devices can provide tremendous benefits to patients, but they can also pose risks. As a regulatory agency, the FDA is committed to ensuring that the information about these products that manufacturers and distributors disseminate to patients and providers is accurate and balanced.

The documents represent the FDA's current thinking on specific aspects of its evolving consideration of social media sites and other Internet related matters. The FDA continues to review, analyze, and develop approaches to a variety of topics related to the labeling and advertising of medical products, including the development of these and other guidances addressing the use of social media platforms and the Internet. Note: See more at http://blogs. fda.gov/fdavoice/index.php/2014/06/fda-issues-draft-guidances-for-industry-on-social-media-and-internet-communications-about-medical-products-desinged-with-patients-in-mind/#sthash-.GjNmfUi5.dpuf.

Healthcare Rating Sites

In the era of social media, healthcare provider rating sites are growing. The sites allow patients to post anonymous comments about their providers regarding everything from how long they're kept waiting for appointments to their treatments. Providers argue that they are hampered by confidentiality issues and can't respond to negative online reviews without risking breaching patient privacy rules.

Due to the increasing importance of healthcare rating sites, healthcare providers must manage their online reputations. To do so, they should consider the following recommendations:

1. Take the feedback as objectively as possible.
2. Don't ask patients to post positive reviews or sign agreements stating they won't write negative ones.
3. Rather than ignore negative ratings, consider monitoring what is being said, and take measured steps to deal with these reviews offline.

General Social Media Guidelines

The following are basic guidelines for employees and volunteers who participate in social media. Social media includes personal blogs and other websites, including but not limited to Facebook, LinkedIn, Google+, Twitter, and YouTube. These basic guidelines apply whether employees and volunteers are posting to their own sites or commenting on other social media sites:

1. Follow all organizational policies. Do not share confidential or proprietary information. Patient privacy and confidentiality must be maintained and protected at all times.
2. Write in the first person. Make it clear that you are speaking for yourself and not on behalf of the organization.
3. Include a disclaimer in the personal section of your blog or social media profile. "The views expressed on this website are my own and do not reflect the views of my employer."
4. When communicating on the Internet, disclose your connection and role in the organization. If you identify your organizational affiliation, your social media activities should be consistent with the organization's professional conduct policies and procedures.
5. Be professional, use good judgment, and be accurate and honest in all communications.
6. Make sure that your social media activity does not interfere with regular work commitments.

7. Patient care staff generally should not initiate or accept friend requests from patients, except in rare circumstances such as a situation where a personal friendship predates the treatment relationship.

8. Managers should not send friend requests to employees they manage. Managers may accept friend requests if initiated by an employee, but only if the manager does not believe doing so will negatively impact the work relationship.

9. On social media websites, where the organizational affiliation is known (e.g., LinkedIn), personal recommendations and endorsements should not be given or requested.

10. Unless approved by the organization, your social media name, handle, and URL should not include the organization's name or logo. Always, ask the appropriate supervisor if you have any questions about what is appropriate to include in your social media profile.

Conclusion

Healthcare providers should contact their professional organizations to get more information on using social media. Organizations must develop and disseminate social media management programs. Additionally, healthcare leaders should consider the following four steps when developing their social media management strategy:

- Identify the benefits and risks of using social media in the organization, and develop the best ways to manage those risks.
- Write a social media management plan.
- Develop, enforce, and update social media protocols and procedures to address appropriate and inappropriate use of social media communication methodologies.
- Manage social media according to written organizational protocols and procedures. This is often a shared responsibility between multiple departments, including but not limited to information technology, public relations, marketing, executive staff, supervisors, human resources, and media relations.

7

PHILANTHROPIC DATA MINING

EVERY YEAR MILLIONS of people use their computers and mobile phones to self-diagnose. They put their symptoms into a search engine, and within seconds, dozens of health-related websites appear on the screen. The search supplies both information for the patient and data for those who survey disease outbreaks by monitoring information regarding how people report symptoms. Cell phones, mobile devices, the Internet, and social media have opened a two-way information channel in health research. The Internet provides unlimited information to the public, and at the same time, the public virtually reveals their locations, concerns, opinions, experiences, and movements from one place to another.

This two-way exchange is dramatically influencing disease information surveillance. It supplements the tools available to monitor, inform, and respond to pandemics and disasters. Likewise, it gives research organizations, including pharmaceutical companies, valuable data that can be used to improve the lives of tens of millions of people.

Accuracy studies of how social media platforms cover epidemic health threats are rare. One study, conducted by the consulting firm ICF Macro on behalf of the Agency for Toxic Substances and Disease Registry, found that blog and Facebook postings covering two environmental health issues—perchlorate (used to make rocket fuel) found in baby food and mold problems with drywall from China—matched what appeared in official reports on the same topics. In general, researchers found that what most people said via the Internet was fairly accurate.[54]

This form of "big brother" monitoring is raising concerns about privacy and about how data generated by cell phones and social media should be available to assist healthcare providers and researchers. There is a new movement called data philanthropy in which companies are finding ways to release data for the benefit of population health without risking individual privacy. At all levels, public health professionals and healthcare researchers understand the absolute public health value and potential of getting this data.

To monitor flu outbreaks, the Centers for Disease Control and Prevention (CDC) traditionally relies on outpatient reporting and test results supplied by laboratories nationwide. The traditional system confirms flu outbreaks within two weeks after they begin. However, monitoring tweet streams can alert the CDC to potential areas of concern in real time. Ideally scientists want as much individualized information as they can get to anchor social network predictive models in real world data. The power of these models was illustrated in a 2010 study that found social network analyses can predict flu outbreaks earlier than traditional tracking methods.[56]

Cell Phones

Among the world's 7 billion people, an estimated 5.3 billion have cell phone accounts, and cell phone coverage extends to 90 percent of the global population.[57] Every call made pinpoints the user's location. Thus, cell phones can track mass movements in which a major change from the norm may represent the impact of a disease or a migration away from perceived threats.

Social scientists want to use cell phone information to develop models of social behavior, but cell phone carriers worry about the inappropriate use of customer data and are reluctant to allow scientists access to this information. If health disaster responders were able to have real time access to track post disaster migration, they could find and help large groups of affected people. For example, cell phone data made it possible to track population movements in Haiti after the January 2010 earthquake and during the subsequent epidemic of cholera.

For his research, Bengtsson petitioned Haiti's largest cellular carrier, Digicel, headquartered in Kingston, Jamaica, for access to position data from roughly 1.9 million cell phones in the island nation corresponding to the period extending from 42 days before the earthquake until 158 days after. According to co-author Johan von Schreeb (a surgeon from the Karolinska Institute), Digicel released the data only after company officials were satisfied that, as academics, Bengtsson and his team wouldn't use the information for economic gain.

Results from the study showed that an estimated 630,000 people who were in the Haitian capital of Port-au-Prince when the earthquake struck had left within nineteen days. The major recipient areas of the refugees, according to the phone data, included three coastal towns: Les Cayes on the southern coast; Leogane, east of the capital; and Saint-Marc to the north. In addition, an estimated 120,000 people who were outside the capital prior to the quake moved into the city during the same nineteen-day period. These findings were consistent with a retrospective United Nations survey conducted six months after the disaster, the authors report. Unfortunately for tens of thousands of people, the movement patterns predicted by the phone data were more accurate but far different from the Haitian government's official real time estimates upon which relief operations relied.[58]

To detect changes in population movement and monitor outbreaks, baseline data are needed. But obtaining access to this data poses major hurdles. Companies might be willing to form data-sharing partnerships with health agencies and nongovernmental organizations, assuming that uses are limited to research and charitable causes. Cell phone companies might also allow data access in exchange for analytical services focused on building better models for delivering service to cellular subscribers.

Social networks

Within social networks, people with perceived credibility and access can have a disproportionately larger influence on public opinion.[59] In addition, social media communication networks can interact with and influence one another. For example, when key figures in a communication network (e.g., government health officials, news reporters, and community leaders) raise alarms about a potential disease outbreak or relay information about a new medical breakthrough, social network trends shift as people respond to that information.

Social media platforms have made healthcare communication more democratic. Now, anyone with access to a computer and an Internet connection can transmit health information worldwide. This new global capability can create unpredictable consequences. For instance, parents may refuse to immunize their children because of something they read or heard about online.

Patient Resources

Internet sites and resources have emerged as popular health communication media. Patients, their families, companions, friends, caregivers, and healthcare providers use social media to discuss disease issues, share personal stories, and connect with friends and support networks. Using social media helps patients expand disease related knowledge, find opinions about or validate information received from healthcare providers, and prepare information for provider visits.

Caregivers and families seek specific health information such as alternative treatment options, recent news, diagnostic and prognostic information for validation, and emotional relief. They also find information to assist patients who may not have the technical expertise or the physiological or psychological strength to engage on social media sites.

Not surprisingly, most of the shared medical information in social media is specific to personalized disease matters, often based on one individual's experience with the ailment. Increasingly, however, healthcare professionals also use web-based tools to share clinical knowledge, professional values, and personal experiences.

Social media activity can promote good health as well. In fact, studies on the healing effect of expressive writing, based on the aspect of online social support, have been reported in the oncology social work and psychology literature.[60] Clearly, the Internet and other electronic communication tools are changing the ways patients and providers receive and provide health information and support.

PatientsLikeMe Open Research Platform

PatientsLikeMe is a leader and innovator for crowdsourced patient data and open research platforms. It works with Genentech, a division of Roche Pharmaceuticals, to examine new forms of evidence to improve their business and impact their products and services. PatientsLikeMe has opened up its online data to pharmaceutical companies several times in the past, including working with Sanofi to recruit participants for clinical trials in 2013, and they had a similar arrangement with Merck made in August of 2012.

Past partnerships have all been limited in scope to a particular product or disease area. However, Genentech will have access to PatientsLikeMe's network to enable cross-sectional research and broader discovery of patient insights. The company will be able to search the data set more effectively and start their own research projects on the platform. They will also be able to use PatientsLikeMe's network to inform patients about clinical trials. [61]

Conclusion

Social media presents a double-edged sword for healthcare philanthropic data mining. As a portal for channeling the personal experiences of billions of people, it represents a valuable reflection of our society: the good, the bad, and everything in between. Effectively using data mining could take the protection of public health to a new level.

8

NONPROFIT FUNDRAISING

Social media is unmatched in power and scope by any fundraising methodology that has been developed in the last fifty years.[62] In the area of healthcare nonprofit fundraising, text messaging, Facebook, and Twitter social media campaigns have proven to be powerful tools, raising tens of millions of dollars relatively quickly. The larger, well-known nonprofits with recognizable brands—such as the Susan G. Komen Breast Cancer Foundation and the American Red Cross—have raised large amounts of money using social media. Lesser known healthcare nonprofit organizations have also experienced success raising money through social media.[63]

Social media fundraising should be considered as an active, evolving, long-term methodology rather than a short-term, get-rich-quick source of funding. A large part of fundraising that is done both online and offline is not immediately or directly related to collecting donations. More often than not, social media is used to build relationships to further fundraising goals in the future.

Getting Started
As with any new technology, training staff and volunteers to use social media effectively would be the first and most costly step.

However, since almost everyone has some experience already with social media, initial training costs can be minimized.

While experience is important in fundraising, younger people tend to be adept and open to using online social media tools. Larger organizations can outsource technology and social media training, but smaller businesses could start by using employees who have the most experience and build from there. Additionally, a social media committee could be formed by recruiting a team of skilled volunteers.

Return on Investment

As with any strategic decision, time spent on social media requires a thoughtful return-on-investment (ROI) strategy and a cost-benefit analysis that assesses strengths and weaknesses. The ROI assessment can be complex and not easy to quantify. There is no simple solution. However, when doing social media fundraising, organizations should ask the following questions:

1. Is social media leading to increased giving?
2. Is social media reaching a larger audience and increasing the prospective donor base? If yes, by how much?
3. Is social media increasing the donor conversion rate? If yes, by how much?
4. Is social media decreasing the cost per donation?

These ROI questions are essentially the same as would be applied to any fundraising strategy. The difference is that with a printed newsletter, the cost can be determined in terms of time, printing, staff, and mailing and measured against the money received, new donors, new prospects, and new clients. In comparison, using social media, someone reads the post, comments on it, and tweets or e-mails it to another person or group. In turn, these other people can "like" it, repost it, and so on. The difference in using social media over traditional fundraising is that social media offers the possibility of limitless interactions. Social media–based fundraising puts more value on interactivity than traditional fundraising, which seeks a direct response.

The ultimate goal is to convert increasing numbers of prospects into donors, and the major role of social media is to positively impact the nonprofit agency's fundraising efforts over time. It does not provide a quick fix, nor should an immediate ROI be anticipated.

Let's say a nonprofit healthcare organization's mission is to research the effectiveness of using social media to positively impact patient health outcomes. Through the limitless boundaries of the Internet, this message can identify and reach patients, bloggers, influencers, families, physicians, academics, researchers, students, other nonprofit organizations, pharmaceutical companies, and thought leaders directly concerned with this issue. At the same time, on a broader scale, the nonprofit can simultaneously connect with the National Institutes of Health and its centers within. As the nonprofit posts, tweets, blogs, or becomes part of a conversation, it continually builds its organization's public brand and elevates the credibility of the agency and its cause. This also lays the groundwork for future fundraising.

A social media strategy requires a paradigm shift from traditional fundraising. Traditional proprietary, self-serving thinking needs to change to what is commonly referred to as "open source." Instead of having a secret giving strategy, social media nonprofits need to share, compare, and expose their work and ideas to like-minded individuals and groups. By sharing, a nonprofit organization is not only spreading its ideas but also gathering constructive criticism and furthering its message and mission.

Social media has chipped away at the foundation of traditional donor-engagement models. Until recently, the models that nonprofits used to find, engage, and cultivate donors, volunteers, and other supporters were reasonably straightforward. The first step was to use direct mail, phone calls, or other techniques to bring in large numbers of potential supporters at a low level of engagement. Supporters were sorted into groups, and the most promising were continually moved up the ladder and cultivated for larger donations. It was an orderly and linear process.

The Internet and social media have permanently disrupted this process. Online competitions, viral video campaigns, mobile giving, and many other new ways for organizations and donors to interact have become increasingly complex methods of donor engagement. They offer greater variation in movement along the pathway to deeper engagement and more opportunities for a person to be influenced by forces outside an organization's control.

Donor behavior and nonprofit communication methodologies have changed drastically due to social media. As a result, traditional donor-engagement models are no longer sufficient. In their place is a new model of donor engagement, one that is more fluid and continuous. This new social media–based model reflects the growing importance that an individual's influence has in the process of increasing contributions.

Traditional Donor-Engagement Model

Ladders have traditionally been used as organizing models in the donor-engagement process. This system was relatively simple: donors exist at a single level at a given point in time and progress up the rungs through carefully calculated outreach and engagement. On every level, greater efforts are made to encourage donors to increase their financial commitments.

Donors at the bottom are less engaged than those nearer to the top. Contributors at different levels take different actions and donate in differing amounts. Thus, different communication tools are associated with each level. Limited touch and automated tools like direct marketing are at the bottom, and more time and labor intensive communication tools like personal outreach are reserved for high end contributors.

In the traditional donor-engagement model, the majority of people enter at the bottom. There is an initial period in which a person gets to know the organization and the organization gets to know the person. At the beginning, the organization may ask the person to get involved in some small way, such as by volunteering for an event, forwarding an email to friends, or signing a petition.

Then, they may ask for a small financial gift. This is followed by stewardship and deeper engagement, further research into the person's capacity to give, and eventually a request for a larger donation. In theory, the cycle continues until a contributor reaches the top of the ladder.[65]

Social Media's Impact

The traditional ladder models have persisted into the new age of social media, as organizations try to make sense of how to use these new tools and determine what advantages, if any, they hold for fundraising. Nonprofits can't ignore the power of social media for fundraising as ever-increasing numbers of people use social media channels to network and gather and process information.

The approach many nonprofit organizations have taken is to integrate social media into the traditional ladder models. Social media is used to help develop and recruit contributors on the bottom rungs, build awareness, and foster relationships through engagement. It is not often used as a way to engender or demonstrate real depth of commitment. "Liking" a cause on Facebook, blogging or tweeting about it, or adding an organization's logo to a personal social profile is considered surface-level (bottom rung) action.

The goal, of course, is to move the casual social media user up the ladder to become a legacy donor. However, the pathway a social media contributor would take and the best way to use the new mix of online, offline, mobile, and social media tools are still a mystery to many organizations. A bigger question is whether social media is the best use of a person's or organization's time and resources for fundraising.

Despite efforts to combine the old and new, there is an inherent disconnect between the static ladder models and the dynamic ways in which people interact with causes today. That is why a new model of donor engagement needs to be developed. To start, it's important to better understand the changes in how donors engage with organizations and causes today.

Healthcare organizations, of course, should not abandon traditional means of donor outreach and engagement in favor of Twitter, YouTube, and Facebook. But a person's engagement with an organization is now different and more complex because of social media and changing technologies. Due to virtual engagement possibilities, engagement doesn't stop and start with discrete levels. With the broad range of activities available to potential supporters, it's preferable to engage people on multiple levels.

Communication Changes

In the same way that, in most cases, traditional funding models no longer represent donor behavior, healthcare nonprofit organizations are too often using outdated donor communication. Today's donor communication models should encourage the segmentation of communications strategies like social media, e-newsletters, and other automated channels at the bottom and personal outreach, face-to-face meetings, and other labor-intensive channels at the top. Segmented communications strategies are blurring in a world where the boundaries between offline and online, traditional and nontraditional forms of communication intersect.

The most successful nonprofit fundraising organizations will be those that embrace strategies integrating online and offline channels. Future success is about creating all-encompassing, multichannel strategies using various media in people's everyday lives that increase opportunities to introduce and reinforce organizational messages. Direct mail and newsletters can be valuable methods of disseminating information, but the power of social media is its ability to provide continuous, timely, and increasingly expanding communications.

The traditional communication models also fall short because they are inherently one way: going from the organization to the person. A person's commitment to an organization can depend on many factors that are outside the organization's control. The friends, family, and peers of donors can greatly influence actions and deepen commitment. Additionally, donors can influence their peers. Organizations need to recognize that they are not always the best messengers. Fundraising professionals and organizations accustomed to operating under one-dimensional models that do not take into account the variable nature of peer-to-peer influence are at a significant disadvantage.

Creating a New Model

Given what is known about the shortcomings of the traditional donor-engagement models, it is possible to construct the outline of a new social media–based model that takes into account changes in donor behavior, communications, and potential outside influences. The new model should incorporate the following characteristics of donor engagement:

- Donors and potential donors are engaged at different levels using multiple communication methods, and as individuals, they can choose to move between the levels.
- Donors and potential donors are never excluded from the engagement process.
- Donor needs, not the organization needs, represent the center of the engagement.
- Donor management understands and accounts for the influence of other people on the strength of the donor-organization relationship.

Adopting this new model will require organizations to change the way they think about their donors and potential donors, and how they assign value and ask for contributions from these groups. It also requires organizations to change the ways in which they train and empower their employees to engage with stakeholders.

Redefining Contributions

The first change a nonprofit organization needs to make is in how it defines and values a person's contribution. Although the ladder models tend to emphasize a singular call to action (i.e., donate money), a new model should value other types of contributions like retweeting a message, "liking" a Facebook page, or subscribing to a YouTube channel.

When organizations emphasize financial donations as the primary means of support, they may be discouraging other types of activities that could significantly expand the reach and influence of the organization. The most valuable people to an organization may be social influencers who post, retweet, and rate an organization and encourage other people to donate. Now, with social media, it may not be the direct donors who have the most value; it may be supporters who can virtually expand the organization's message to reach tens of thousands of potential donors.[66]

For a nonprofit, a valued supporter could be a small donor with a high social media presence, or a higher degree of social platform expertise, who can influence others to give well beyond their own capacity. Where the traditional models might write this person off as not worth an organization's time and investment, a new model that takes influence into account will give that person a much higher value.

Diversifying Calls to Action

Once an organization begins to define and value contributions differently, it can diversify its calls to action. If organizations believe financial donations are the most important level of involvement, they are losing the opportunities that would come by asking supporters to share online message appeals with their personal networks. Supporting a cause by spreading the message is relatively easy, requires minimal effort, and can develop into substantial benefits.

Americans recognize the value of social media for promoting causes. Because there are so many different activities in which people become involved, healthcare nonprofit organizations must think more strategically about what they ask from their supporters. To better understand the relative importance of different types of activities, they can be categorized in two dimensions: level of involvement (e.g., personal investment in time and resources) and level of influence (e.g., how likely completing an activity will lead to others getting involved).

Donating money, for example, has a relatively high level of involvement, assuming it represents a reasonably substantial contribution, but a low level of influence if a person donates and tells no one about it. Forwarding an email to friends about a cause has the potential to influence other people to get involved, giving it a high influence value but a lower value for involvement because it's a relatively easy task.

Sustaining Continual Communication

The way to meet the challenge of staying in continual communication with donors is to encourage more people in the organization to help. Most organizations train board members to deliver basic elevator speeches. To take full advantage of social media, nonprofit organizations need to embrace the "everyone is a communicator and organizational representative" philosophy.

Ongoing organizational communications and content generation can also be enhanced by supporters. Online supporters can be identified, trained, and managed like any group of volunteers. A few minutes on the organization's Facebook page would reveal people who are consistently posting, reposting, and liking organizational posts. These are the people who can be recruited to become online content-creation ambassadors.

Due to an expectation of losing control, some nonprofit organizations may hesitate to empower external ambassadors. There's some concern that these ambassadors will not appropriately deliver the organization's message. However, most issues have two sides. With the loss of some control, there may come an increase in down-to-earth, relevant, transparent, and authentic communication that can greatly enhance a brand. [67]

Go4theGoal Seasonal Lace Up 4 Pediatric Cancer Campaigns

During September, Pediatric Cancer Awareness Month, Go4theGoal worked exclusively with Akron Children's Hospital's Development and Media Relations team to promote its Lace Up 4 Pediatric Cancer® campaign throughout the Akron region. With Lace Up 4 Pediatric Cancer®, youth, high school, college, and professional sports teams purchased Go4theGoal's gold shoelaces and gear to wear during a special childhood cancer awareness game. Funds generated from sales of laces as well as any additional donations stayed local to help support those affected by childhood cancer. The initiative raised an estimated $40,000 in just one month.

Ice Bucket Challenge

The Ice Bucket Challenge is the latest trend to take social media by storm. Participants dump buckets of ice water on their heads and post videos of it on social media sites, challenging their friends to do the same within twenty-four hours. They also use the hashtag #IceBucketChallenge to help spread the word and raise funds for ALS, also known as Lou Gehrig's Disease. From July 29, 2014, to August 14, 2014—approximately two weeks— the ALS Association received $9.5 million from donors.

Conclusion

Social media has changed the ways in which people can influence others and increased the range of meaningful calls to action available to nonprofits. Continual communication is now an expectation, if not a demand. The full impact of these changes on the traditional donor-engagement models is in flux. However, it is clear that new ways of thinking about donor behavior should incorporate measures of influence and better account for dynamic and fluid ways in which people support causes. Even as influence continues to be defined, organizations can respond to these shifts by rethinking their definitions of a contribution and diversifying their calls to action. The challenge is finding ways to maximize the contributions of different groups of people with unique desires and resources.

9

CROWDSOURCING

CROWDSOURCING COMBINES THE wisdom and resources of a diversified group of individuals, usually via the Internet, who offer ideas, comments, resources, and solutions. It is basically a model for groups of people to help healthcare organizations fund projects, improve innovation, manage information, and analyze data. Small healthcare businesses are using crowdsourced funding for projects, major brands are crowdsourcing advertisements, and start-up businesses are crowdsourcing logos.

Despite endless layers of regulation, the challenges currently faced by healthcare providers, patients, and researchers make crowdsourcing a potentially effective tool to initiate collective problem solving. The Internet's democratization and collaboration can assist information-dependent professionals who use crowdsourcing to increase quality of care, needed resources, and innovation.

Healthcare crowdsourcing often takes the form of open innovation initiatives, in which organizations promote external appeals for ideas. For example, InnoCentive (http://www.innocentive.com/) helps companies and nonprofits issue global challenges that invite people to propose solutions to problems. The best submissions receive prizes ranging from $5,000 to $1 million.

With the impending pay-for-performance changes in reimbursement, the healthcare system will be challenged to keep expenses down and increase quality while dealing with an aging population. In a world of cost and time constraints, crowdsourcing can be an excellent new tool for organizations.

InnoCentive works extensively in the healthcare field, partnering with pharmaceutical companies, advocacy groups, and medical centers. In the last decade, its healthcare-related challenges have yielded significant advances, including the identification of a biomarker for the nonprofit Prize4Life as well as an algorithm for predicting cancer survival rates for the Cleveland Clinic.[75]

Using only traditional innovation methods, an organization can spend years pursuing one of many possible solutions, only to reach a dead end. Crowdsourcing can bring hundreds, if not thousands, of people together to pursue multiple potential solutions. Then, organizations need pay an award only for solutions that prove to be productive.

Crowdsourcing changes the economics, statistically increases the potential for finding a better solution, and can result in innovative outcomes that never could have been anticipated. Crowdsource outcomes offer unlimited potential for the healthcare industry. Possible outcomes could include discovering treatments or cures for thousands of diseases, learning how to use social media to positively affect patient outcomes, minimizing the spread of HIV for at-risk youth, and start-up funding for an innovative healthcare product or service.

Crowdsource Patient Information (PatientsLikeMe)
Social networking sites, such as PatientsLikeMe, gather individuals with specific health conditions so they can share and compare their symptoms and responses to different treatments. In 2012, PatientsLikeMe unveiled its open research exchange platform, which allows researchers to develop, test, and conduct surveys.

PatientsLikeMe, a social network, is producing some of the most compelling clinical data the healthcare industry has ever seen. PatientsLikeMe was launched in 2004 by family members of a man who had contracted ALS five years earlier at the age of twenty-nine. They raised millions of dollars in a failed effort to find a cure for ALS, and at the same time, they created a data-sharing patient social network to go with it. PatientsLikeMe now has more than two hundred thousand patients on the platform and is tracking eighteen hundred diseases.

Crowdsourcing Disease Surveillance

Public health experts are using crowdsourcing as a faster alternative to traditional methods for predicting and monitoring infectious disease outbreaks. For instance, in Haiti in 2010, informal sources such as news reports, discussion groups, and Twitter noted a cholera outbreak two weeks before the health ministry issued its official report. Public health projects like NCB-Prepared and HealthMap analyze data from both formal and informal sources—including World Health Organization alerts, local health departments, news sources, and social media—to detect disease outbreaks and provide real-time surveillance.[75]

Crowdsourcing Health Innovation

Healthcare innovation using crowdsourcing methodologies is a dynamic process through which problems and challenges are defined, new and creative ideas are developed, and new solutions are selected and implemented. It is a coordinated, complex process with many layers and feedback opportunities. Crowdsourcing is a deliberate, learning-based method that brings about qualitative and quantitative results using unconventional wisdom.

Innovation could include identifying, translating, and adapting new global ideas and solutions to problems in the United States. Thus, crowdsourcing may not always provide original, unique solutions; the information may include programs that have worked in other countries.

Public Health Crowdsourcing

For years, for-profit corporations have asked their customers what they want. Business social media and websites are filled with requests for customers to help develop new products, new flavors and choose the latest advertisements. Now is the time for public health to use proven crowdsource communication methods employed in the private sector and ask for help from the people they serve.

The rate of data being generated about healthcare, patients, population health, interventions, technology, and research far outpaces the ability of individuals to keep up with it. Crowdsourcing can be used to find, evaluate, decipher, and recommend information that may be lost in. the nearly unlimited access to data and healthcare information overload. For instance, professionals can use crowdsourcing to solve a problem by posting the issue on an appropriate LinkedIn group and requesting solutions from group members.

There are many sources of innovation in the public health sector. Digital technologies offer new opportunities for reorganizing the interaction between underserved patient populations and public health authorities, and technology breakthroughs challenge the form and content of public health services.

Elected politicians, healthcare policy experts, public health managers, and citizen groups are requesting innovative solutions to the problems and challenges of improving population health. Public health departments can clearly articulate problems and then use crowdsourcing to request innovative opportunities and possible solutions, mobilize resources, and exploit windows of opportunity.

Crowdsourcing innovation can be further enhanced by bringing together influential members of a target population who can identify and define problems and challenges in ways that capture their complexity. Then, this carefully selected target group could develop new strategies and solutions for dealing with unique circumstances. Targeted groups can offer ideas that take into account the potential risks and benefits of innovative solutions, and the group can help to determine the best course of action. Finally, the actualization of the new plan can be facilitated by the originating influential group, who can now take joint ownership of the solution, implementation, and resolution.

Using collaborative crowdsourcing methodologies in the public sector ensures that public health innovation draws upon and brings into play relevant assets in terms of knowledge, imagination, cultural competence, creativity, resources, transformative capacities, and powerful local influential capabilities. Collaborative crowdsourcing is a major paradigm shift for traditional public bureaucracies that exchange resources and ideas within their organizational and institutional borders.

Collaborative innovation can also be enhanced by connecting public health officials in one region to similar professionals throughout the United States. These geographically connected groups can collaborate to inform, educate, develop, and test new solutions.

Healthcare Crowdsource Funding

Healthcare venture capitalists are always looking for the next blockbuster. Crowdsource funding is now available to help small entrepreneurs raise money to develop healthcare inventions and bring them to market. Entrepreneurs and small developers are rushing to crowdsource funding sites to subsidize their new healthcare technologies. Entrepreneurial healthcare providers, technically astute healthcare administrators, and peripheral healthcare suppliers are using crowdfunding sites to finance their projects. Crowdsource funding offers access to money, expertise, and an immediate measure of marketability. In 2012 crowdsourced funding generated $5 billion in investment for healthcare apps and devices.

In the past, healthcare inventors used personal funds, loans from friends and family, and credit cards to finance their projects. Now, using crowdsourcing, inventors can mix funding approaches. Recipients only have to worry about getting funded and paying a nominal charge to the site.

10

CONCLUSION

THE RAPID EVOLUTION of technology has transformed society. The growing capacity to store, analyze, and transmit information allows behavioral, social, and medical data to be combined to help detect the spread of disease and support treatment, education, and health promotion. Mobile Internet platforms offer opportunities to coordinate community healthcare services, and mobile technologies empower consumers to manage their own health. Given the tremendous growth of mobile technology and social media communication, the positive impact on health is only limited by what can be imagined.

Doctors, patients, and public health and government officials are suffering from information overload. It is not humanly possible to stay current with all the changes in healthcare. Thus, the healthcare industry is like a runaway train with no breaks. Blink, and something new, something major, something dramatic, something that will change healthcare forever was just introduced. One idea is to stop blinking and live in a delusional world believing all this chaos is a fad.

As the commercial world goes social, the social-based business of healthcare is not far behind. Social internal networking enterprise tools can be leveraged to improve coordination of care among healthcare professionals; streamline the development of clinical content; enable distributed research teams to accelerate drug discovery; enhance customer service between health insurers and their members; and advance staff training, learning, and continuing medical education within the workplace. This list represents a few examples emerging every day in a rapidly expanding healthcare internal social networking environment. There is little doubt the world of healthcare internal enterprise social networking and collaboration will continue to become more prevalent in the coming years.

Many older academics, healthcare professionals and administrators, public health officials, and government leaders who are in positions to make high-level decisions may not be nor want to become computer literate. These power brokers can certainly continue to stick their collective heads in the sand, but like it or not, healthcare is changing. Healthcare is going digital, and it is happening now. To prepare the next generation for this inevitability, digital literacy must be an important part of all healthcare training and education programs worldwide.

Communication affects all patients and healthcare professionals. Thus, social media will become more important within healthcare, but balance is needed. E-patients should not ignore the value of their healthcare professionals, just as healthcare professionals should not ignore the power of the Internet to engage their patients. Healthcare providers, public health professionals, and healthcare administrators must join the digital movement or expect to become obsolete. We are at the very beginning, and the healthcare digital world is rapidly moving forward.

Many older parents and grandparents are becoming more heavily engaged in social media channels. The new era of healthcare demands that all providers engage with their patients and families when, how, and where the customers desire. For many patients and families, the first touch point with an organization will be with a digital platform (e.g., website, social channel, etc.). It is important to make patient interactions easy and professional, whether it be in helping customers learn more about services, find a provider, or request an appointment. This is the starting point for long-lasting patient-provider relationships.

Creating social media channels is essential. They contribute to customer loyalty and positive word-of-mouth recommendations, which is increasingly important to a brand's reputation. Providers should take the time to assess each channel to determine their target audience and the appropriate content. For example, science and research content receives higher engagement through a LinkedIn company page, whereas a strong patient story will be better placed on Facebook.

Providers must understand their patients in order to engage them and their families, and it is important to provide an enhanced patient experience through digital platforms. Regardless of the channel, providing compelling content is key, and providers should always strive to stay true to this requirement. They must treat social media as an integral part of the patient experience and work to create a supportive, inspirational, and informative environment for past, current, and prospective patient families. Patients and their families have never been more involved in their own care and the care of their loved ones, so it is essential that providers start to use social media to communicate with their patients and their families.

People search the Internet for information, for meaningful connections, reviews, support systems, and advocacy. By sharing patient success stories and offering advice, tips, and health information, providers will create a dynamic environment that is a useful resource for patients and families. Providers need to respond to each question, demonstrate that they are listening, direct patients to the care they need, and celebrate customer milestones, such as healthcare achievements, birthdays, and graduations.

It is important to measure engagement levels with the links shared through social media channels and blogs. By tracking clicks and page views, time spent on pages, and so on, providers will have a better sense of which content is and isn't working. While social media can sometimes be difficult to track and analyze, providers will need to measure results, continue to make changes, and move forward in a positive direction.

Online engagement is becoming more mobile based. There are many tasks users can now accomplish on mobile devices that could not have been done in the recent past. As the healthcare industry shifts to an online presence, there will be more of a need to meet a mobile-first patient mindset.

To maximize the online patient and family healthcare experience, providers' websites must be fully responsive, enabling patients and families to find the information they need from any device, anywhere. A website needs to respond to the user's screen size to provide the optimal user experience, whether it be on a desktop, tablet, or mobile phone.

During the next few years, rather than requiring one application to find a provider, another to pay a bill, and yet another to find a location, providers should integrate all activities into one cohesive user experience. Healthcare is changing rapidly, which means opportunities abound. Sophisticated patient communication and engagement have only just begun.

How to Prepare for the Future

The following are seven basic steps for healthcare providers to begin using social media:

- Embrace digital technologies. Use technology to make life easier and work more efficient.
- Influence decision makers to make changes if a specific idea to use new technologies can improve outcomes.
- Be bold and use social media channels to spread the word.
- Use a variety of digital media sources to follow the main trends within a niche, and stay current in an area of expertise.
- Learn what technologies competitors use.
- Be cautious regarding accessing false or misleading information.
- Strategically analyze trends, and plan for the future.

Social media offers so many new possibilities that can be used in the healthcare industry. It can be used for marketing, informing, alerting, inspiring, mentoring, educating, increasing organizational productivity, advancing internal communication, raising money, crowdsourcing, promoting brand awareness, engaging, improving patient outcomes, and researching. It also offers many virtual opportunities for providers and patients to become strategic partners in helping patients make better personal healthcare choices.

Due to access to nearly infinite health information, people using social media sites will be introduced to false or unreliable details. Thus, to help patients make better decisions, providers must be sure to provide accurate content. Using Skype-type programs, telemedicine is becoming a reality. With open access and crowdsourced scientific information, it is possible to conduct clinical trials and research. Crowdsource research can often gather the same amount of information with similar quality as before, but in a much faster, noninvasive, humane, and reliable way.

The number of healthcare mobile applications has been rising exponentially. With so many choices, providers and patients are finding it more difficult to choose the right apps. To get better patient outcomes, providers can create their own mobile apps to include functions like logging blood pressure or medication compliance.

The benefits of using social media in healthcare continue to increase. Emerging platforms have extended the abilities of individuals and businesses to increase communication with peers, family, friends, colleagues, and customers. Social media enhances personal and professional relationships; allows for more efficient exchange of knowledge; creates opportunities for professional interactions; and provides new possibilities to disseminate information and discuss health-related education, research, and best practices.

Organizations have begun to use social media in ways that attempt to meet the demands of their patients, employees, subcontractors, insurers, and the general public. Social media is a significant factor regarding how patients use the Internet for healthcare. Ninety-four percent of twenty-three thousand respondents in the

Pew Report identified Facebook as their primary source for health related information, followed by YouTube. Almost one-third of survey respondents reported their trust in social media as "high" or "very high," and one-quarter reported that the information they find on social media is "likely" or "very likely" to influence their decisions.

Healthcare organizations use social media to raise organizational awareness by sharing corporation news and services, community events, and general news from local or national media. Success stories highlighting staff, healthcare provider, or patient achievements, awards, or struggles drive traffic to the organization's website.

During the Boston Marathon bombing, local hospitals communicated with patients, families, and staff via Facebook, providing information on blood donation and statistics on victims being treated (e.g., number of patients in each condition level), sharing expert advice on coping with the event, and updating staff on scheduling issues. Three hospitals receiving the majority of casualties—Massachusetts General Hospital, Brigham and Women's Hospital, and Beth Israel Deaconess Medical Center—used status updates to notify the community of changes in their security status, operating procedures, and appointment cancellations throughout the week after the bombing. Finally, Boston hospitals used their social networks to thank their supporters and share acts of kindness happening in their facilities. As evidenced by the Boston Marathon tragedy, social media is becoming a major crisis-communication tool.

Potential uses of social media by healthcare organizations include disaster management; blood donation promotion; weight management and support; epidemiological tracking; outpatient appointment arrangement; mentorship; encouragement and support; suggestions and referrals to support and treatment services; arrangements for outpatient care; real-time satisfaction surveys; and food, product, and pharmaceutical safety alerts.

The healthcare industry's reluctance to adopt social media has been driven largely by concern about potential risks of privacy violations, inaccurate information dissemination, and loss of public trust. Patient privacy in the social media age is an evolving issue requiring hospitals to be proactive. Social media distributes information instantaneously to a wide audience, and unlike verbal conversations, it creates a permanent electronic record that cannot be fully deleted and may be used in court proceedings.

When using social media, managing the organization's reputation is one of the most significant risks, second only to privacy protection. The organization must be aware of and respond to criticism and complaints that originate outside the organization and must ensure that social media content accurately reflects the organization's message and does not harm its reputation. To manage an organization's reputation, management practices must include having employees engaged in social media to be aware of what is being said about the organization, provide timely responses, and be respectful in all communications.

Organizations need policies to manage content originating both outside and within them. There are numerous examples of individuals and celebrities doing lasting harm while working on behalf of an organization when they posted crude, inappropriate, or otherwise unprofessional content on social media.[80]

While the number of medical mobile applications has been rising, persuading clients to keep using the apps is a challenge. The question is not whether such applications could be used in the process of practicing medicine or delivering healthcare but rather which ones to use and to what extent they can be helpful. The FDA has issued preliminary guidance that might facilitate the process.

Improving diagnostics and treatments should not be enough anymore. The overall healthcare experience needs to significantly improve. Healthcare delivery must mirror the customer experiences that are common in the hospitality industry. After getting their diagnoses, patients should have access to comprehensive information to help them make better decisions.

The use of social media has expanded networking to facilitate personal and professional relationships; allowed for more rapid exchange of knowledge; created forums for collegial interactions;

and provided for dissemination of information and discussion regarding health-related education, research, and best practices.

Final Note
Social media has great potential for providing information to health-care professionals and consumers. We are beginning to learn that the broader the social network, the greater the opportunity to extend the conversation to new dimensions, making teamwork and care collaboration a seamless effort to engage clinical teams for answers that save lives. The use of social media and the possibilities of social learning networks can improve the care provided. By being careful of the potential ramifications of misusing social media, healthcare providers can enjoy the personal and professional benefits of social media without violating patient privacy and confidentiality. Now is the time for the entire healthcare industry to embrace the use of social media as a new, innovative, essential and valuable form of communication.

REFERENCES

1. *The 2009 H1N1 Pandemic: Summary Highlights April 2009–April 2010*, updated June 16, 2010, accessed Aug. 18, 2014, http://www.cdc.gov/h1n1flu/cdcresponse.htm.

2. Cancer Survivors Network, accessed Aug. 18, 2014, http://csn.cancer.org/.

3. Pew Research Internet Project, accessed Aug. 18, 2014, http://www.pewInternet.org/fact-sheets/health-fact-sheet.

4. "Social Networks in Health Care: Communication, Collaboration and Insights,"
http://www.ucsf.edu/sites/default/files/legacy_files/US_CHS_2010SocialNetworks_070710.pdf

5. Aha Guide 2014 website, retrieved August 31, 2014, http://www.hhnmostwired.com/

6. Deanna Reed, "Using Social Media for Doctor-to-Doctor Communication," July 5, 2012, http://wordviewediting.com/using- social-media-for-doctor-to-doctor-communication/.

7. Angela Haupt, "How Doctors Are Using Social Media to Connect with Patients," Nov. 21, 2011, http://health.usnews.com/health-news/most-connected-hospitals/articles/2011/11/21/how-doctors-are-using-social-media-to-connect-with-patients.

8. David Pittman, "'Meaningful Use' Stage 3 May Increase Patient Interaction," *MedPage Today*, Feb. 19, 2014, http://www.medpageto-day.com/PracticeManagement/InformationTechnology/44395.

9. "Social Media and Healthcare: Navigating the New Communications Landscape,"

http://www.healthcareitnews.com/blog/social-media- and-healthcare-navigating-new-communications-landscape.

10. John Trader, "Social Media and Healthcare: Navigating the New Communications Landscape," June 24, 2013, retrieved August 23, 2014, http://www.healthcareitnews.com/blog/social-media-and-healthcare-navigating-new-communications-landscape

11. Alan Neuhauser, "Health Care Harnesses Social Media," *US News &World Report,* June 5, 2014, http://www.usnews.com/news/articles/2014/06/05/health-care-harnesses-social-media.

12. Christopher A. Cassa et al., "Twitter as a Sentinel in Emergency Situations: Lessons from the Boston Marathon Explosions," *PloS Currents*, July 5, 2013, doi: 10.1371/currents.dis.ad70cd1c8bc585e9470046cde334ee4b. See more at http://journalistsresource.org/studies/government/criminal-justice/boston-marathon-bombings-research-lessons#sthash.Yvo8d161.dpuf.

13. Rick Burnes, "Inbound Marketing & the Next Phase of Marketing on the Web," *HubSpot*, November 18, 2008, http://blog.hubspot.com/blog/tabid/6307/bid/4416/Inbound-Marketing-the-Next-Phase-of-Marketing-on-the-Web.aspx.

14. Kurt Wagner, "Facebook Passes 1 Billion Monthly Mobile Users," *Mashable*, April 23, 2014, http://mashable.com/2014/04/23/facebook-1-billion-mobile-users/

15. Neal Cabage and Sonya Zhang, "Web 3.0 Has Begun," *Interactions,* September–October 2013, http://interactions.acm.org/archive/view/september-october-2013/web-3.0-has-begun.

16. Barb Dybwad, "Google Reader Adds Magic to Your Feeds," *Mashable,* October 22, 2009, http://mashable.com/2009/10/22/google-reader-personalization/.

17. Robin Wauters, "LinkedIn Acquires mSpoke for Its Recommendation Technology, Team," *TechCrunch*, Aug. 4, 2010, http://techcrunch.com/2010/08/04/linkedin-mspoke/.

18. Stuart Dredge, "How Does Facebook Decide What to Show in My News Feed?" *Guardian*, June 30, 2014, http://www.theguardian.com/technology/2014/jun/30/facebook-news-feed-filters-emotion-study.

19. Wen-ying Sylvia, Chou, Yvonne Hunt, Ellen Burke Beckjord, Richard P. Moser, Bradford W. Hesse, "Social Media Use in the United States: Implications for Health Communication," *Journal of Medical Internet Research,* November 27, 2009

http://www.ncbi.nlm.nih.gov/pmc/articles/PMC2802563/.

20. Clarissa Schilstra, "The Patient's Perspective on Social Media in Healthcare," *Medical Practice Insider*, July 15, 2014, http://www.medicalpracticeinsider.com/best-practices/patients-perspective-social-media-healthcare.

21. Daniella Koren, "Patient Engagement: It's More Than You May Think," *Media Post,* March 31, 2014, http://www.mediapost.com/publications/article/222576/patient-engagement-its-more-than-you-may-think.html.

22. CMS.gov, "Meaningful Use Stage 2: Regulations and Guidance," http://www.cms.gov/Regulations-and-Guidance/Legislation/EHRIncentivePrograms/Stage_2.html.

23. Judith Hibbard and Jessica Greene, "Engaged Patients Translate to Better Outcomes and Costs," *The Healthcare Blog*, Feb. 10, 2013, http://thehealthcareblog.com/blog/2013/02/10/engaged-patients-translate-to-better-outcomes-and-costs/.

24. V. J. Strecher et al., "Goal setting as a strategy for health behavior change," *Health Education Quarterly*, 22, no. 3 (1995): 410, http://www.ncbi.nlm.nih.gov/pubmed/7622387.

25. Emory University; David Bray, Karen Croxson, William Dutton, and Benn Konsynski, "Sermo: A Community-Based Knowledge Ecosystem," OII-MTS Case Study, Version 6.0, January 2008, http://www.emory.edu/BUSINESS/readings/ecosystems/SermoBriefing.pdf.

26. Ricardo De Leon "Scoop It: Social Media, Youth and Health Literacy," http://www.scoop.it/t/social-media-youth-and-health-literacy.

27. "Report: Interactive Monitors Help Boost Patient Satisfaction," *Healthbeat,* Thursday, March 10, 2011, http://www.ihealthbeat.org/articles/2011/3/10/report-interactive-monitors-help-boost-patient-satisfaction.

28. Peter Murray, "Survey: 78 percent of patients believe EHRs boost care," *Healthcare IT News,* March 8, 2011.

29. Elizabeth Smith, "Is Social Media the Way to Reach the Teenage Patient?" *JHU Communication Career Blog,* http://jhucommunication.wordpress.com/2014/06/20/is-social-media-the-way-to-reach-the-teenage-patient-by-elizabeth-smith/.

30. Jenn Francis, "Tech-Savvy Seniors Seek Digital Tools to Manage Health, According to Accenture Survey," /19/2014 newsroom.accenture.com/news/tech-savvy-seniors-seek-digital-tools-to-mange-health-according-to-accenture-survey.

31. Aetna, "Healthcare Professional RelayHealth FAQs," http://www.aetna.com/faqs-health-insurance/health-care-professionals-relayhealth-faqs.html.

32. John Bradley Jackson, "Baby Boomers: Excessively Selfish or Proudly Individualistic?" http://www.firstbestordifferent.com/blog/?p=1542.

33. Jim Gilmartin, "Marketing to Baby Boomer and Senior Customers," *Media Post,* January 7, 2013, http://www.mediapost.com/publications/article/190455/marketing-to-baby-boomer-and-senior-customers-pa.html.

34. Ann Carrns, *New York Times,* "Health Care Apps Offer Patients an Active Role," April 25, 2014, http://www.nytimes.com/2014/04/26/your-money/health-care-apps-offer-patients-a-more-active-role.html?_r=0.

35. Kim Komando, "Apps to Help People with Alzheimer's," *USA Today,* June 14, 2013, http://www.usatoday.com/story/tech/columnist/komando/2013/06/14/brain-fitness-app-email-accounting-software-charity/2407599/.

36. Joan Patterson, "Smartphone Apps Let Patients Gauge Entry Times for Emergency Rooms," *Las Vegas Review Journal,* January 12, 2014, http://www.reviewjournal.com/life/health/smartphone-apps-let-patients-gauge-entry-times-emergency-rooms.

37. Stacey Patterson, "11 Super Mobile Medical Apps," *Information Week,* http://www.informationweek.com/mobile/11-super-mobile-medical-apps/d/d-id/1105143?

38. Jacques Bughin et al., "The Social Economy: Unlocking Value and Productivity through Social Technologies," McKinsey & Company, July 2012, http://www.mckinsey.com/insights/high_tech_telecoms_internet/the_social_economy.

39. Ali H. Al-Badi et al., "Usage of Social Networking Tools in Research and Collaboration," *Journal of Emerging Trends in Economics and Management Sciences* (JETEMS), 4, no. 6 (2013): 515–23, http://jetems.scholarlinkresearch.com/articles/Usage%20of%20Social%20Networking.pdf.

40. Nichole Kelly, "Using an Internal Social Network to Solve Real Business Problems: The Opportunity Your Company Could Be Missing," *Social Media Explorer,* October 8, 2013, http://www.socialmediaexplorer.com/social-media-marketing/using-an-internal-social-network-to-solve-real-business-problems/.

41. Felice Espiritu, "The Evolution of an Open Innovation Tool," *Kaiser Permanente IdeaBook*, 2011, http://www.cimit.org/images/events/ciw102511/IdeaBook_FeliceEspiritu_102511.pdf.

42. David Kiron, "Using Social Tools to Improve Customer Service, Research and Internal Collaboration," *Big Idea: Social Business Interview*, March 6, 2012, http://sloanreview.mit.edu/article/kaiser-permanente-using-social-tools-to-improve-customer-service-research-and-internal-collaboration/.

43. Eric Savitz, "5 Ways Social Media Will Change the Way You Work in 2013," *Forbes,* Dec. 11, 2012, http://www.forbes.com/sites/ciocentral/2012/12/11/5-ways-social-media-will-change-the-way-you-work-in-2013/.

44. Tibbr Admin, "How Fortune 100 Companies are Flattening Hierarchies Through Enterprise Social," http://www.tibbr.com/blog/topics/enterprise-social-network-topics/why-are-leading-organizations-turning-to-a-flatter-organizational-hierarchy/.

45. Business Dictionary, http://www.businessdictionary.com/definition/privacy.html#ixzz3A0kCA1f9.

46. Investor Words, http://www.investorwords.com/13093/confidentiality.html#ixzz3A0lHDtFC.

47. Margaret Rouse, "Data Protection," *WhatIs.com,* http://searchstorage.techtarget.com/definition/data-protection.

48. Marlene M. Maheu, Myron L. Pulier, and Frank H. Wilhelm, *The Mental Health Professional and the New Technologies* (Mahwah, New Jersey, Taylor & Francis, Sep 18, 2004), 230. The Mental Health Professional and the New Technologies: A Handbook for Practice Today Hardcover – July 22, 2004

49. HHS.gov, Health Information Privacy (1966), http://www.hhs.gov/ocr/privacy/index.html.

50. Brian Honigman, "24 Outstanding Statistics and Figures on How Social Media has Impacted the Healthcare Industry, 2013, http://community.advanceweb.com/blogs/nurses3/archive/2014/07/16/does-social-media-have-a-place-in-healthcare.

51. *Steven M. Harris,* "How to Avoid Data Breaches, HIPAA Violations When Posting Patients' Protected Health Information Online," *The Hospitalist,* June 2014, http://www.the-hospitalist.org/details/article/6203581/How_to_Avoid_Data_Breaches_HIPAA_Violations_When_Posting_Patients_Protected_Heal.html.

52. *Healthcare attorney Anne P. Schmidt is based out of the Philadelphia office of Burns White and represents clients throughout Pennsylvania. She can be reached at* apschmidt@burnswhite.com.

53. "Internet/Social Media Platforms with Character Space Limitations: Presenting Risk and Benefit Information for Prescription Drugs and Medical Devices," Draft Guidance, June 2014, http://www.fda.gov/downloads/Drugs/GuidanceComplianceRegulatoryInformation/Guidances/UCM401087.pdf.

54. "Guidance for Industry Internet/Social Media Platforms: Correcting Independent Third-Party Misinformation About Prescription Drugs and Medical Devices," Draft Guidance, 2014

http://www.fda.gov/downloads/Drugs/GuidanceCompliance Regulatory Information/Guidances/UCM401079.pdf.

55. The research was presented at the American Public Health Association's 2011 Annual Meeting.

56. Christakis Na et al., "Social Network Sensors for Early Detection of Contagious Outbreaks," *PLoS ONE* 5, no. 9 (2010): e12948, http://dx.doi.org/10.1371/journal.pone.0012948.

57. ITU. *The World in 2010: ICT Facts and Figures* (Geneva, Switzerland: International Telecommunication Union, 2010), accessed Dec. 12, 2011, http://www.itu.int/ITU-D/ict/materiai/FactsFigures2010.pdf.

58. L. Bengtsson et al., "Improved Response to Disasters and Outbreaks by Tracking Population Movements with Mobile Phone Network Data: A Post-Earthquake Geospatial Study in Haiti," *PLoS Med,* 8, no. 8 (2011): e1001083, http://dx.doi.org/10.1371/journal.pmed.1001083.

59. Patrick Dunleavy, *Democracy, Bureaucracy and Public Choice: Economic Approaches in Political Science* (New York, New York: Taylor and Francis, 2014).

60. Sujin Kim, "Content Analysis of Cancer Blog Posts," *Journal of the Medical Library Association*, 97, no. 4 (2009): 260–66, http://www.ncbi.nlm.nih.gov/pmc/articles/PMC2759160/#__ffn_sectitle.

61. Jonah Comstock, "PatientsLikeMe Signs Five-year Data Access Deal with Genentech," *Mobil Health News,* April 10, 2014, http://mobihealthnews.com/31960/patientslikeme-signs-five-year- data-access-deal-with-genentech/.

62. John Kania and Mark Kramer, "Nonprofit Management: Collective Impact," *Stanford Social Innovation Review*, Winter 2011, http://www.ssireview.org/articles/entry/collective_impact.

63. Barbara L. Ciconte and Jeanne Jacob, *Fundraising Basics: A Complete Guide* (Bolingbrook, IL: Jones & Bartlett Learning, 2011).

64. Ken Burnett, *Relationship Fundraising: A Donor-Based Approach to the Business of Raising Money* (NY: John Wiley & Sons, 2002).

65. Alan Andreasen and Philip Kotier, *Strategic Marketing for Nonprofit Organizations* (Upper Saddle River, NJ: Prentice Hall, 2007); Joe Garecht, "The 5 Steps of Donor Engagement," *Fundraising Authority*, http://www.thefundraisingauthority.com/donor-cultivation/donor-engagement.

66. Paul Smith and Ze Zook, *Marketing Communications: Integrating Offline and Online with Social Media* (Philadelphia: Kogen Page, 2011), 17.

67. Julie Dixon and Denise Keyes, "The Permanent Disruption of Social Media," *Stanford Social Innovation Review*, 11, no. 1 (Winter 2013).

68. B. S. Fjeldsoe, A. L. Marshall, and Y. D. Miller, "Behavior Change Interventions Delivered by Mobile Telephone Short-message Service," *Am J Prev Med.*, 36, no. 2 (2009): 165–73, doi: 10.1016/j.amepre.2008.09.040.

69. Health Resources and Services Administration Department of Health and Human Services, http://www.hrsa.gov/publichealth/healthliteracy/healthlitabout.html.

70. Donya Currie, "More Health Departments Nationwide Embracing Social Media: Use of Tools Rises," *Nation's Health,* http://thenationshealth.aphapublications.org/content/42/4/1.2.full June 2012.

71. James W. Holsinger, Jr., F. Douglas Sctchfield, David M. Lawrence, *Contemporary Public Health: Principles, Practice, and Policy,* (Lexington, Kentucky: University Press of Kentucky, 2012).

72. *The Affordable Care Act: Section-by-Section.* http://www.hhs.gov/healthcare/rights/law/index.html.

73. *Federal Health Information Technology Strategic Plan 2011–2015*, http://www.healthit.gov/sites/default/files/utility/final-federal-health-it-strategic-plan-0911.pdf.

74. Jennifer Cohen,"HealthBizDecoded;How CrowdsourcingFuels Healthcare Innovation,"June 4, 2013, http://www.healthbizdecoded.com/2013/06/how-crowdsourcing-fuels-healthcare-innovation/.

75. Rumi Chunara, Jason R. Andrews, and John S. Brownstein, "Social and News Media Enable Estimation of Epidemiological

Patterns Early in the 2010 Haitian Cholera Outbreak," *Am. J. Trop. Med. Hyg.,* 86, no. 1 (2012): 39–45, doi:10.4269/ajtmh.2012.11-0597; http://healthmap.org/documents/Chunara_AJTMH_2012.pdf.

76. "PatientsLikeMe and Actelion to Develop New Patient-Reported Measure for Mycosis Fungoides-Type Cutaneous T-Cell Lymphoma (MF-CTCL)," posted August 5, 2014 by patientslikeme, http://blog.patientslikeme.com/tag/paul-wicks/.

77. Alison Diana, "Crowd Source Funding," *Information Week.*

http://www.informationweek.com/healthcare/leadership/crowdfunding-the-next-healthcare-hit/d/d-id/1141654.

78. Kristin Lanning, "Physician Engagement: The Next Health Care Social Media Frontier?" Oct 3, 2014. American Hospital Association Health Forum

79. Todd Wilms, "The Overlooked: Social Media Marketing for Senior Citizens," *SAP Forbes,* May 20, 2013.

80. Suby Crys Marie "Social Media in Health Care: Benefits, Concerns, and Guidelines for Use," *Creative Nursing,* Vol. 19, No. 3 (July 1, 2013) Labor Management Institute

Printed in Great Britain
by Amazon